looking**younger**

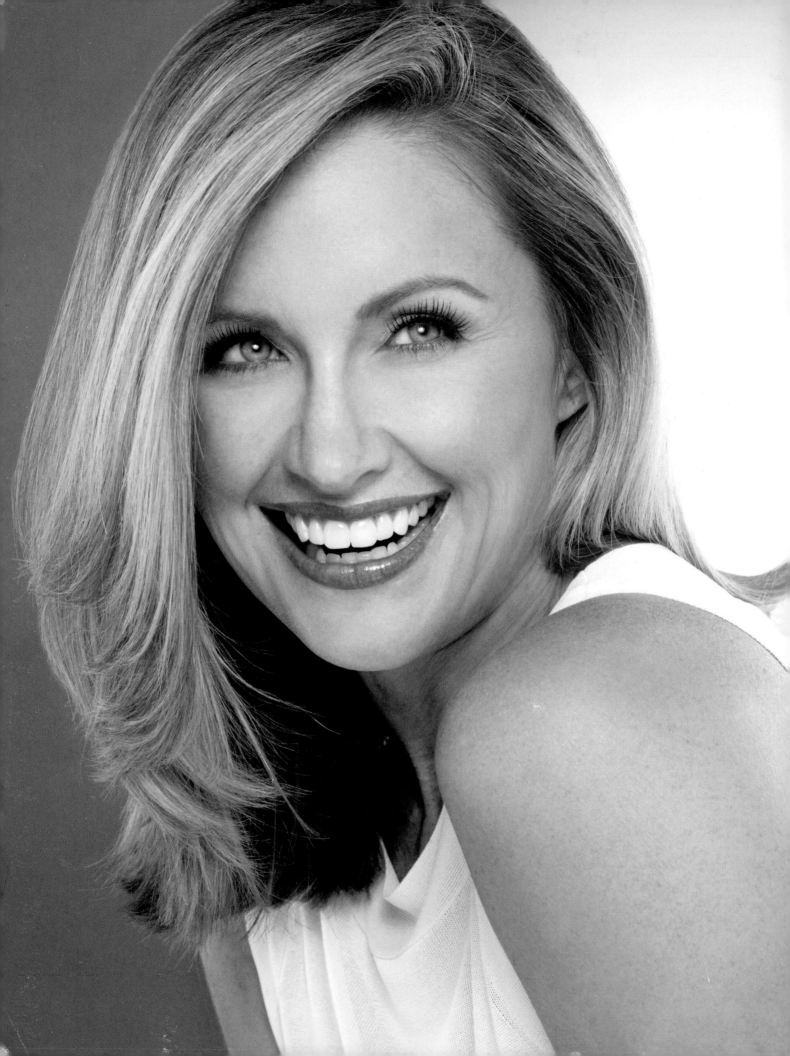

lookingyounger

makeovers that make you look
as young as you feel

beauty

robert jones

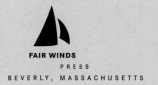

FAIR WINDS
PRESS
BEVERLY, MASSACHUSETTS

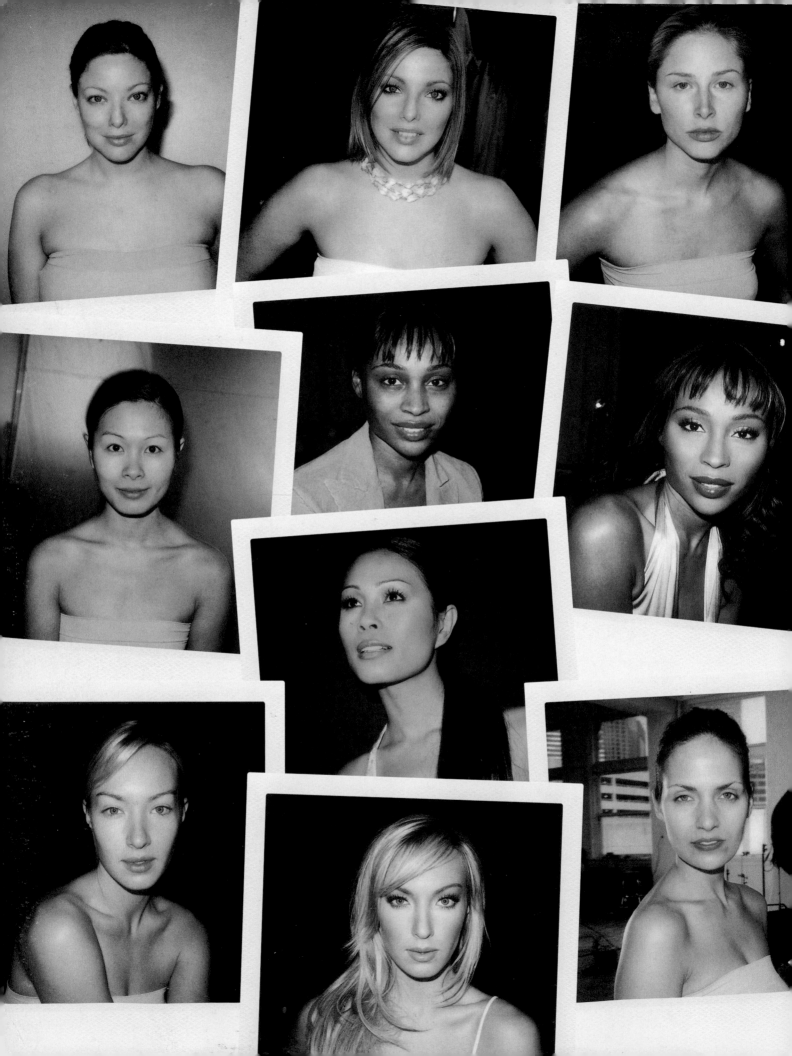

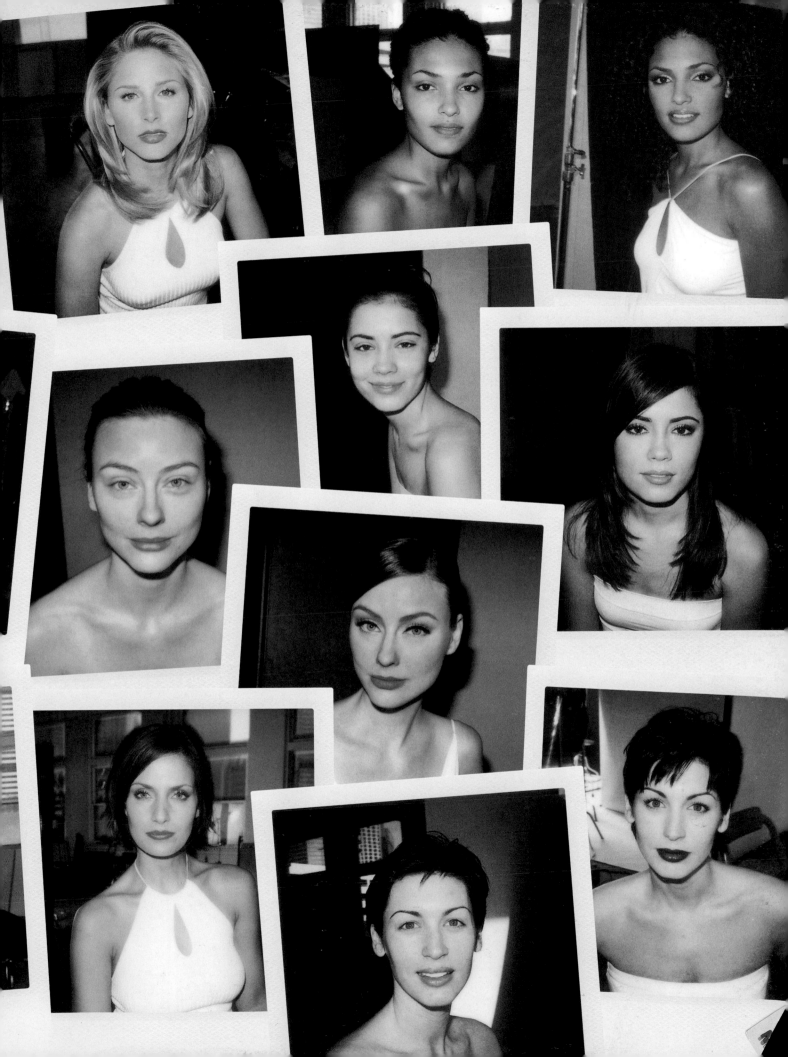

Text and photography © 2008 Robert Jones

First published in the USA in 2008 by
Fair Winds Press, a member of
Quayside Publishing Group
100 Cummings Center, Suite 406-L
Beverly, MA 01915

12 11 10 09 08   1 2 3 4 5

ISBN-13: 978-1-59233-317-2
ISBN-10: 1-59233-317-6

Library of Congress Cataloging-in-Publication Data
Jones, Robert.
    Looking younger : makeovers that make you look as young as you feel /
Robert Jones.
          p.   cm.
    ISBN 1-59233-317-6
    1. Cosmetics--Popular works. 2. Beauty, Personal. 3. Women--Health
and hygiene. I. Title.
    RA778.J6254 2008
    646.7'2--dc22
                              2008007486
Cover design: Carol Holtz Design
Book design: Laura H. Couallier, Laura Herrmann Design
Hair and makeup: Robert Jones, with hair assisted by Missy Brumley,
  Susie Jasper, Stephanie Carranza, Lisa Williams, and Ashley Bell
Representation: Seaminx Artist Management, www.seaminx.com
Production: Elaine Moock, Sunni Smyth, and Patty Woodrich
Fashion and beauty photography: Jeff Stephens
Fashion styling: Patty Flores, Deborah Points, Chad Curry, and Barri Martin
Still-life photography: Fernando Ceja
Still-life styling: Phillip Groves and Linda Jantzen
Illustrations: Robin Kachantones

special thanks to all the women in my life who have inspired and will inspire me
special thanks to Dr. John Morehead, M.D., F.A.C.S. for his talent and expertise
special thanks to everyone at Fair Winds Press that helped make all this happen,
  especially Daria Perreault who saw my vision and understood my craziness, and
  Will Kiester, who put up with my meltdowns. thank you everyone!
www.robertjonesbeauty.com

Printed and bound in China

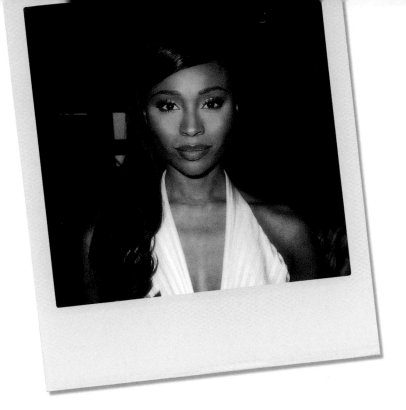

This book is dedicated to all the people who never let me give up. They believe in me, I think, more than I believe in myself. They love me unconditionally and are there to pick me up when I feel like I can't go on. Carolyn Scoville, my grandmother; Chip McFadin, the love of my life; Missy Brumley and Mayolo Gonzalez, the best cheer-leaders ever; Jeff Stephens, without whom this book would not exist. I love you all and am blessed to have and have had you in my life.

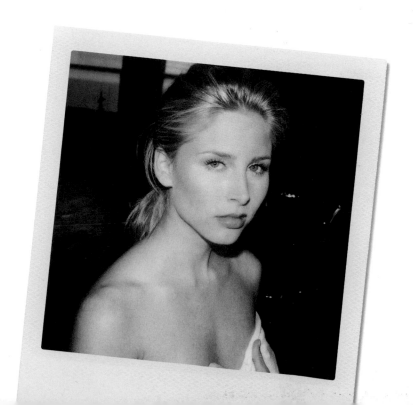

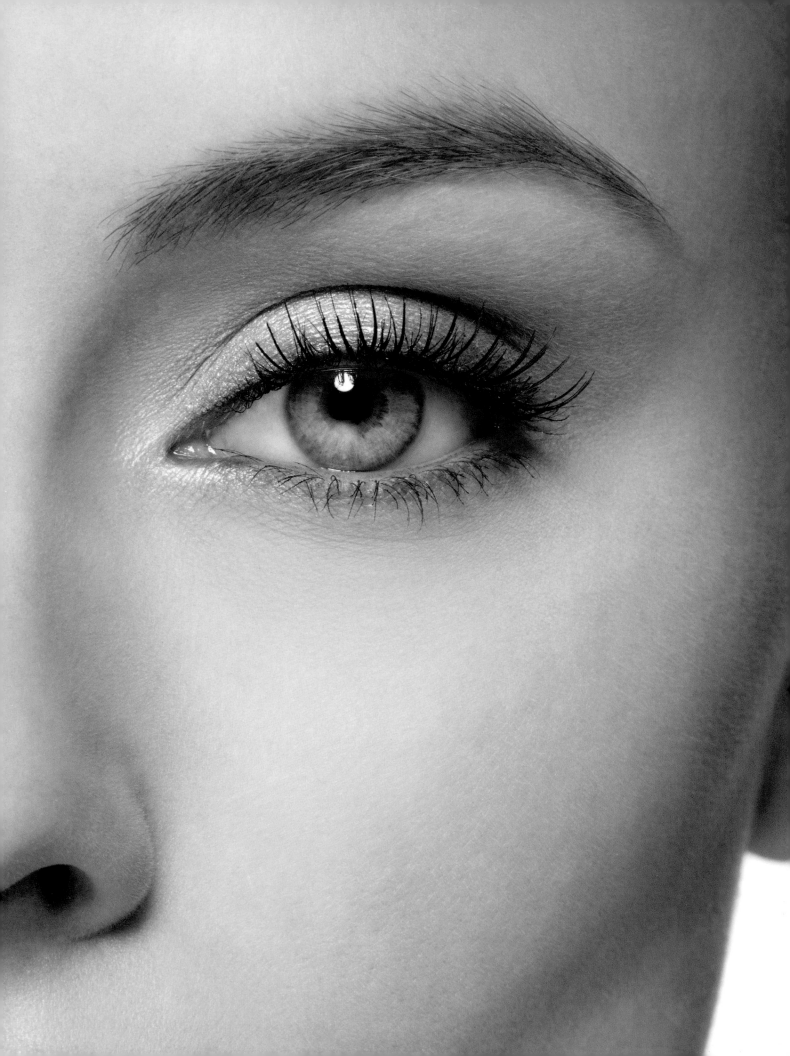

"self-confidence is the
most important element of
true beauty—at any age"

contents

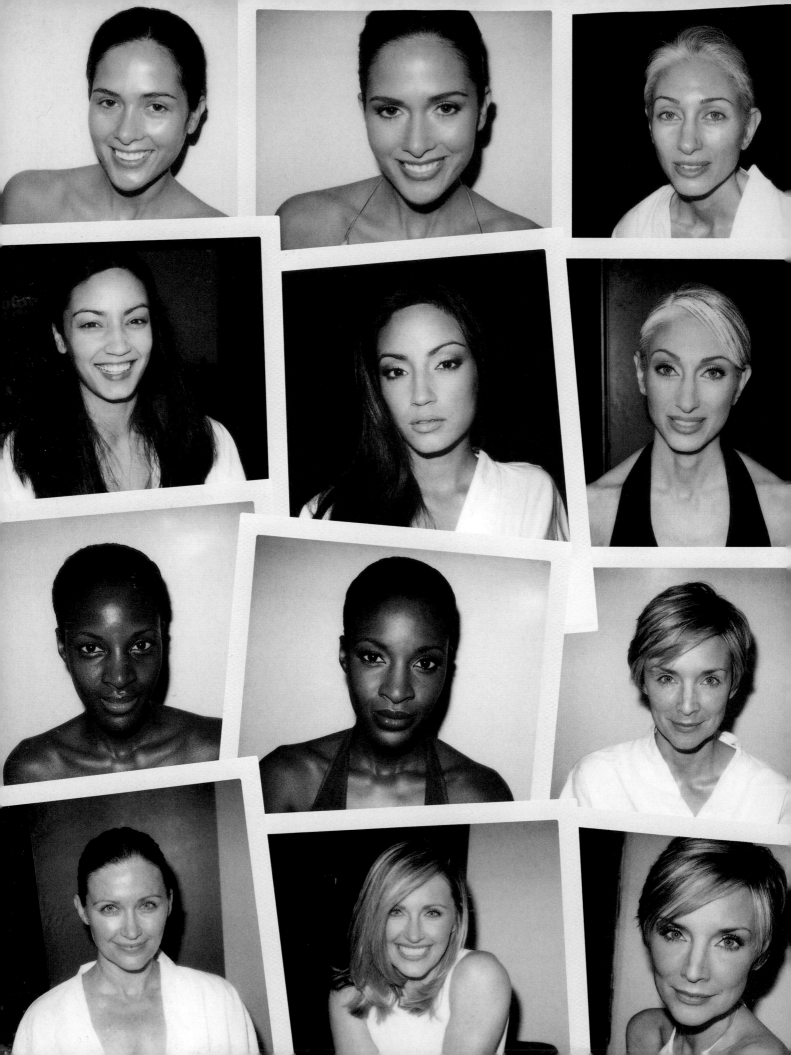

part one | the basics
of looking younger

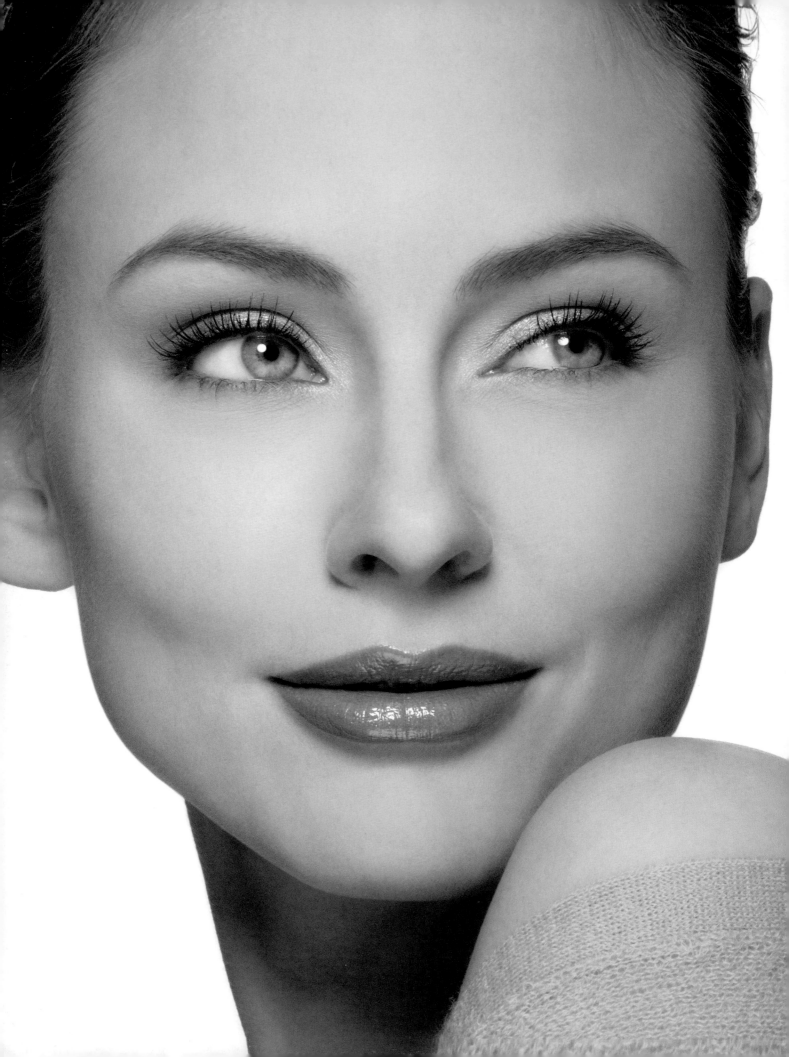

1

what is beauty?

What is true beauty? This can be a hard question to answer, because beauty truly is in the eyes of the beholder, and everyone's truth can be and probably is different.

I could start by making a list of the women I feel have inspired my ideal of beauty. First are the ever-so-expected ones, like Audrey Hepburn, with her polished elegance (especially in *Breakfast at Tiffany's* and *Funny Face*), and Marilyn Monroe, with her sexy vulnerability. (When she appeared on the screen, you couldn't help but look at her; in *How to Marry a Millionaire*, for example—I dare you not to look!) And let's not leave out Elizabeth Taylor, with her strength, beauty, and presence. (I will never forget the first time I saw *Giant* on the big screen; the minute she appeared, she took my breath away.)

But interestingly enough, my strongest beauty influence, as far as famous actresses go, is Barbra Streisand (watch her in *Funny Girl*—she is absolutely mesmerizing). Her awkward beauty and confidence is breathtaking. I look at what I consider to be beauty perfection today, and I can see her influence: a dark, defined eye with shadow that elongates up and out, a softly flushed coral cheek, and a soft, subtle, slightly nude (but not bare) mouth.

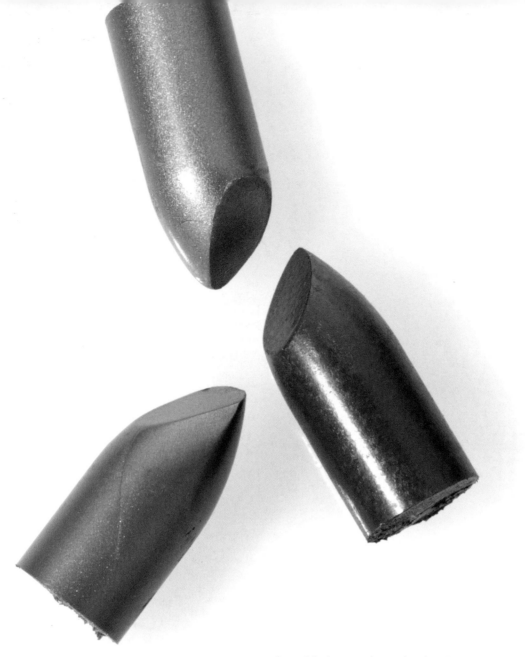

I could also go down the (probably boring for most) list of iconic models that greatly influenced me. The first was Jean Shrimpton. Even today, when I see a photo of her, I am blown away by her beauty and presence (those brows, that mouth, her strong square jaw). Kim Alexis is a perfect example of what the '80s was all about; her looks demand your attention. And then there's the classic beauty of Christy Turlington (gorgeous but still approachable).

I wonder what my appreciation of these women says about my ideal of beauty. Am I too concerned with the superficial, exterior aspect of beauty? This brings me back to the original question: What is true beauty? As I think about this, I have to say that the person most on my mind is my grandmother.

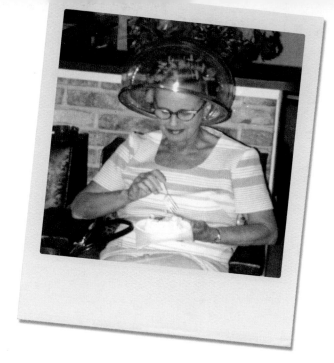

beauty from the inside out

My grandmother was not a perfect beauty—by society's standards, at least—yet she had a presence: She commanded your attention when she walked into a room. Glamorous in her own quirky way—brows too dark, lipstick too frosty—she never left the house without her makeup. She was strong, loving, loyal, predictable. I know those must sound like strange adjectives to use to describe true beauty, but for me, they do. I am flooded by thoughts of all the strong, loving women in my life, and as I think of them, I know that real beauty is having the ability to love unconditionally. I believe that real women are the definition of true beauty: loving, caring, sharing, and being there for those they love.

In working on this book, I shared with my friend, Sandra, my panic about starting the project. She sent me a few thoughts that she felt would help bring my ideas about beauty into sharper focus. I'd like to share them with you, too.

"It is widely believed that most people are obsessed with outward beauty, to the degree that they ignore their inner beauty," Sandra wrote. "They focus on what they look like versus who they are. However, it is possible that the outward expression of someone's beauty is actually a desire to express her inner self.

"Every time I talk with you, I am struck with your genuine desire to get to know people. Is it possible that you are searching for their inner beauty… their kindness…so that you can most effectively express it? You always take the time to make models feel comfortable; you draw them out, you allow them to feel OK about expressing their vulnerabilities. In essence, your artistry is not just an outward persona of beauty but instead an authentic expression of the beauty, kindness, or charm you discover in people as you go.

"I was struck yesterday as we were flipping through your book, that you *knew* each person, and you knew something deeply personal about each woman you had worked with. You speak of them as friends, rather than as subjects. I believe that is what allows you to work at a level unsurpassed by most.

"Think about the role your genuine desire to connect with people plays in your approach and how it allows their inner beauty to surface. I think that is your real talent, and I love you!"

Did Sandra have an insight that I had overlooked? Or was I just not aware of my real feelings about the question of what is true beauty? No—she was just able to express it better than I could.

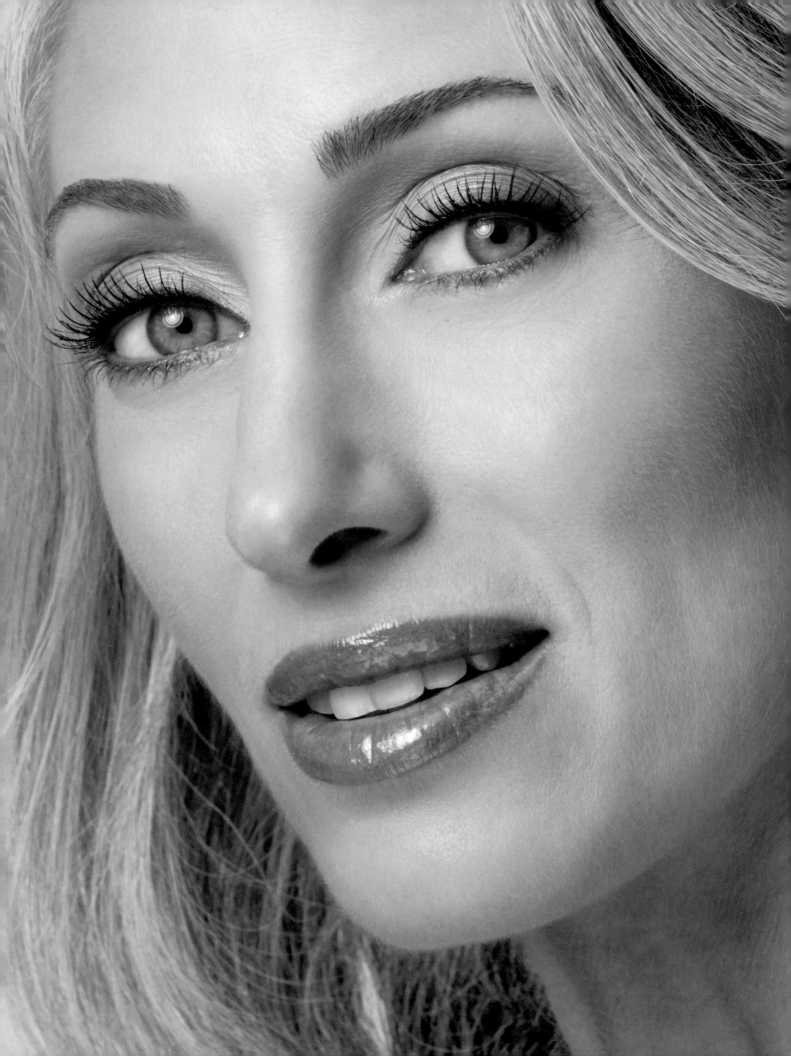

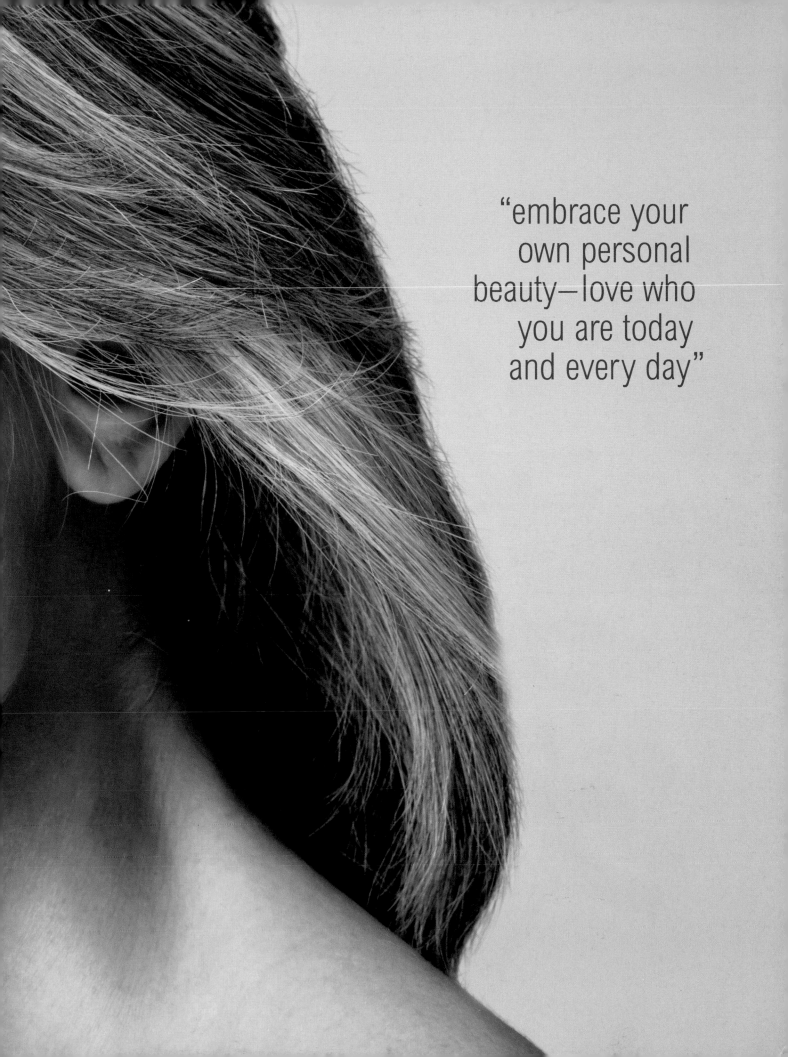

"embrace your
own personal
beauty—love who
you are today
and every day"

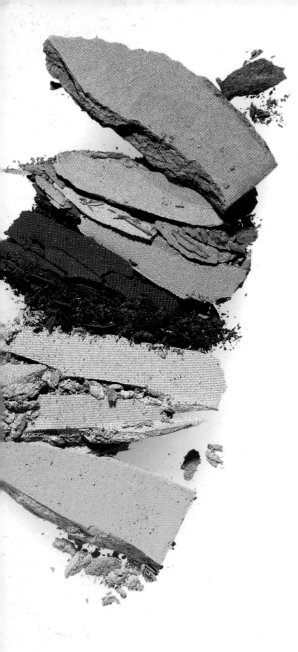

true beauty at any age

For me, true beauty is inner beauty, strength, and a commanding, larger-than-life presence. However, I know that it's hard for many women to let their inner beauty show if they don't feel confident about their outer beauty. So outer beauty does have value; it is not completely shallow. Giving yourself that feeling of confidence is worth spending the effort on your appearance.

Even as my grandmother aged, she took the time to polish her outer beauty, so that her inner beauty could show through. Looking back, I wish I could have educated her with the facts and given her advice (and yes, sometimes just my personal opinions) about *looking younger,* the information that I am about to share with you. Using many of my *looking younger* techniques would have made her an even stronger force to be reckoned with.

The character—the life—in a woman's face is what makes her truly beautiful, the beauty that comes with years of living and, more importantly, loving. You do not want to erase the features that make you who you are! But you can soften those things on the outside that you do not want to see and that are keeping your inner beauty from shining through.

I know many women in their forties and fifties who are truly the most beautiful they have ever been in their lives, because they are living and loving. These women are making choices that help them look radiant and beautiful—not to look twenty. Looking younger is more about looking your most beautiful, regardless of what or where you are in life, than it is about turning back the clock.

The journey to true beauty starts by taking care of your body and skin and continues with bringing your best features into focus. Take that journey with me now, a journey to discover your inner youth and beauty by creating your perfect outer beauty. We will make choices together and learn applications that will arm you with the knowledge you need to find the most beautiful you. Look in the mirror and see the beautiful woman that you are right now. Together, we are going to make you the most beautiful you that you can be.

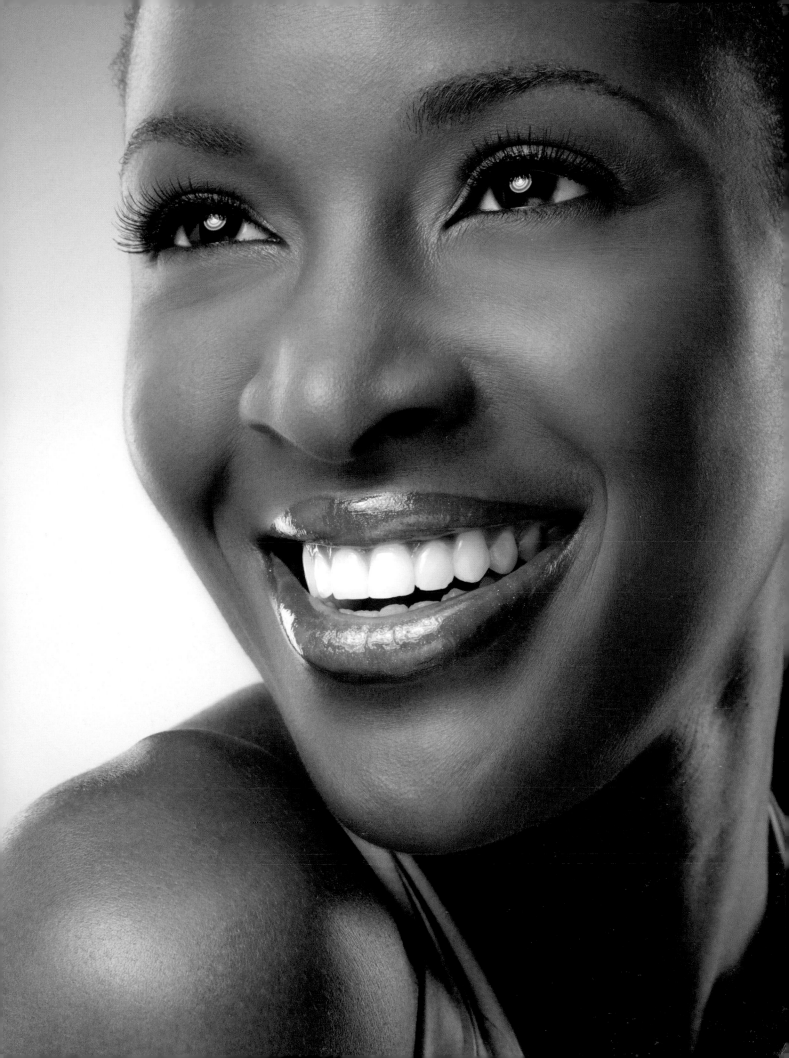

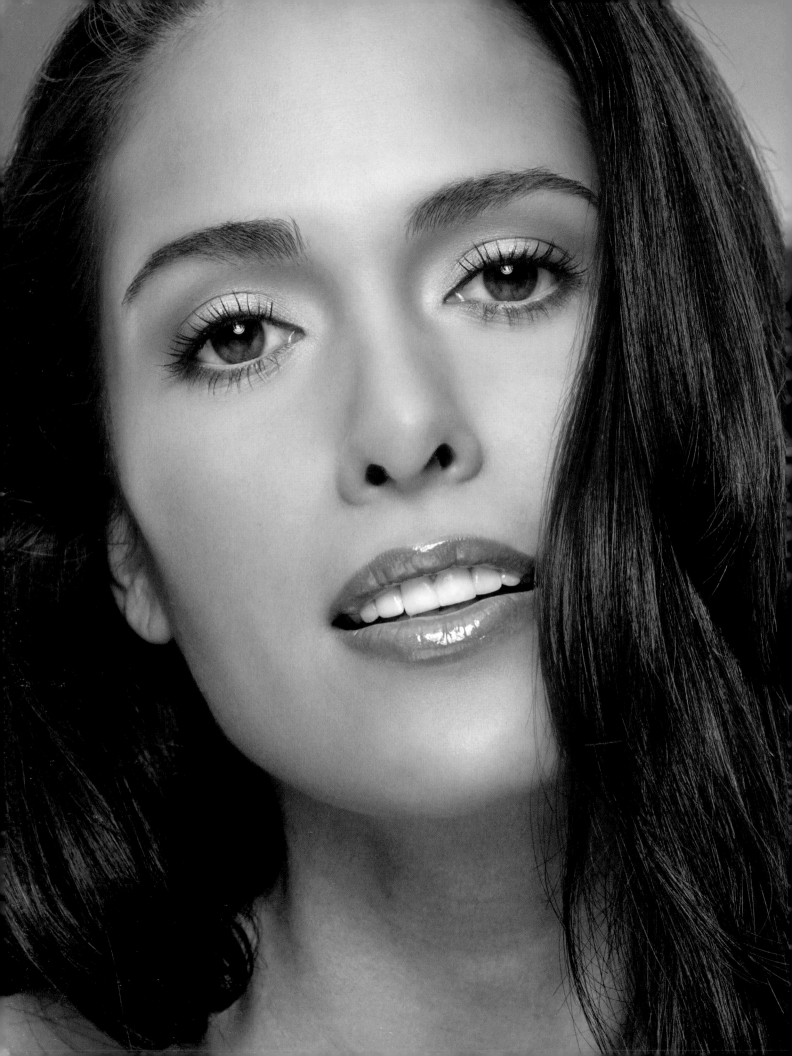

2

what's in a word?

My goal with this book is to help you learn as
much as possible. To help you really understand
all the fine details of makeup and its application.
First I'd like to review with you some key words
that I will use throughout the book. Knowing these
words will greatly enhance what you take away
from our looking younger journey. Although these
are common words in the makeup world, they are
not as common in real life. Get to know and understand them, and you'll be able to ask for—and
find—exactly what you need.

alkaline is the opposite of acidic, in terms of your skin's chemistry. Your skin's pH (the level of alkalinity versus acidity) can affect or change the appearance of pigments in makeup. Your goal with your skincare is to help keep your skin's pH balanced.

antioxidants are nutrients, or ingredients, such as vitamin E, vitamin C, and beta-carotene, which are thought to protect body cells from the damaging (aging) effects of oxidation. They help keep skin looking younger.

apple of your cheek is the full, round, fleshy area of the cheek, which becomes more prominent and is accentuated when you smile.

blot is to remove oil or moisture with an absorbent material, such as blot paper or tissue.

blotchy refers to an unevenness of the skin's tone and appearance. Spots, blotches, and skin discoloration age your appearance.

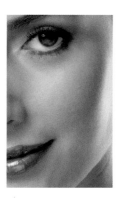

blush adds a wonderfully warm glow to the face and can brighten the dullest of skin. If your cheeks are naturally rosy, you might skip the blush and leave the glow to Mother Nature. But for most, blush can definitely make you look younger.

brighten means to lighten or perk up: for example, to brighten the skin or lip color.

brow bone is the area of the eyelid directly below the arch of the brow. It really is a bone and is more or less prominent, depending on the shape of your skull and eye socket.

capillaries are tiny blood vessels throughout the body and face that connect arteries and veins.

Capillaries form an intricate network around body tissues to distribute oxygen and nutrients to the cells and remove waste substances. When damaged (broken), they show up as thin red lines on the face, commonly around the nose and in the cheek area.

cakey describes a product that appears thick, dry, flaky, crusty, and dehydrated when applied. For example, your concealer can look cakey if applied too thickly or if you use a formula that is too dry for the area to which you are applying it.

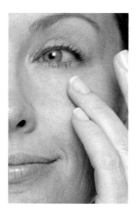

concealer is a miracle product that hides everything your foundation doesn't. Use it to make broken capillaries, under-eye circles, age spots, and skin discolorations disappear. Because its consistency is thicker than foundation, it gives great coverage.

contour is the opposite of highlight (see page 24). Unlike highlighting, which draws the eye to a feature, contouring (or deepening) pushes the eye away from a feature and makes it appear less visible. A "contour shade" is usually a darker shade that gives your features more depth and definition by contrasting them against the lighter shades used on your face and around the eyes. Contouring is also the last step in the three-color layering technique for the eyes (see page 127 for application instructions).

contrast is the brightness ratio of the lightest to the darkest shade. For example, a light eyeshadow is in high contrast to a dark eyeshadow.

crepe-like appearance is when an area of skin appears to have many fine lines and looks slightly saggy; for example, when your eyelids appear to be wrinkled and saggy from excess skin.

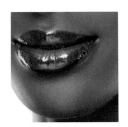

cupid's bow of the lip is the rounded, curved area at the center of the top lip, forming a shape much like an M. Some lips have a more defined bow than others.

dehydrated means to suffer from loss of moisture. Dehydrated areas of the skin lack moisture and suppleness, making them appear older.

depth level describes the lightness or darkness of something, such as skin and foundation. It is how light or how dark your skin and foundation appear to the naked eye.

dewy often refers to a foundation, blush, or lip color whose finish creates a fresh and glowing look, with a slight sheen and luminosity.

discoloration describes an area of skin that has changed from its natural color. These can be dark circles, age spots, and any area of the skin that has changed from your natural skin tone, usually becoming darker, but sometimes lighter, in color.

dual finish refers to products that provide multiple finishes when they're applied. Depending on the application tool you use, you will get either more or less coverage.

elasticity describes the skin's suppleness and its ability to remain firm, taut, and visually tight and youthful. Loss of elasticity, which can be caused by many circumstances, including sun damage, age, dehydration, and genetics, allows the skin to sag, which makes it look older.

emollient is an ingredient that helps smooth and soften the skin and, when added to products, allows them to be pressed into a cakelike form. For example, adding an emollient to a powder allows it to be pressed into a compact and hold together.

exfoliate is the process of using products and actions that slough off or remove the dead surface layer of skin from an area of your body or face, revealing fresh, younger-looking skin.

eyeliner is used for defining and "bringing out" the eyes, though it is not always necessary. It is the product most commonly used to draw attention to the eyes.

eyeshadow can be applied lightly as a gentle color wash or as a more dramatic layering of color and texture to enhance and add shape to the eyes.

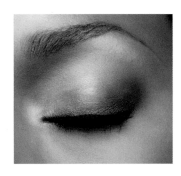

facial masking describes a visible unevenness to the color of the skin. It is particularly visible in bronze/ebony skin, when the innermost part of the face is drastically lighter than the skin of the outer area, creating a dark masked area around the outside of the face.

finish is the appearance a product gives to the surface to which it is applied. Eyeshadows have matte, shimmer, satin, or frosted finishes; lipstick finishes can be matte, crème, shimmer, or frosted.

foundation is a miracle product that evens out your complexion and covers imperfections. Your foundation's tone depends entirely on your skin. If your skin is looking radiant and beautiful without help, then by all means skip the foundation and simply use a light dusting of powder. However, if you do need foundation, you'll find it in a variety of finishes, such as matte, satin, and dewy. If your skin is oily or blemished, choose matte. If your skin is normal or dry, you can choose from any of the finishes.

fragrance-free refers to a product formula to which no fragrance ingredients have been added. This does not mean the product has no scent, because some of its ingredients can have a natural residual smell, giving the product a distinctive scent. But no fragrance ingredients have been added to a formula that states it is fragrance free.

frost is about maximum sparkle and super-shine. It is also sometimes referred to as iridescent. It is a fun, sexy look that works best on young skin, because it can draw attention to the fine lines of mature skin. The term is usually used in reference to eyeshadows and lip colors.

gloss is a super-high-shine lip color. It can add a punch of color but does not stay on as long as lipstick. It will make lips look fuller and younger.

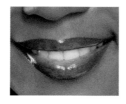

glow means to create a radiance that seems to come from within. A beautiful glow can immediately create the appearance of a youthful radiance that removes years. Glow does not mean shiny, which suggests oiliness and accentuates skin texture flaws; it means radiant and youthful. It is most often created by choosing the perfect shades and textures of foundations, bronzers, and blushes.

highlight is the opposite of contour (see page 22). Highlighting draws attention to a specific area or feature and makes it appear to come toward you. Used on the face and eyes, a highlight shade is usually a lighter shade. Highlighting is the first step in the three-color layering technique for the eyes and is the lightest shade in sculpting the face.

hyperpigmentation is a common, usually harmless, condition in which patches of skin become darker in color than your normal skin color. This darkening occurs when an excess of melanin, the brown pigment that produces normal skin color, forms deposits in the skin.

hypoallergenic cosmetics are products that manufacturers claim produce fewer allergic reactions than other cosmetic products. Consumers with hypersensitive skin, and even those with "normal" skin, might find these products to be gentler to their skin than non-hypoallergenic cosmetics.

hypopigmentation is the loss of skin color. It is caused by melanocyte depletion—a decrease in the amino acid tyrosine, which is used by melanocytes to make melanin, the brown pigment that produces normal skin color.

intensity is a term used to describe the vividness of a product, how strong its shade or color appears. For example, an intense lip color will be very noticeable and attention-grabbing.

layering means to apply multiple layers of a product or products one on top of the other. This technique creates a greater depth of color and also provides more complete coverage of a product.

light-reflecting particles are the tiny, finely ground particles (ingredients) in a formula that reflect light. By reflecting light, they help to disguise flaws that lie underneath. Products with these ingredients work well for creating the illusion of flawless skin without heavy coverage.

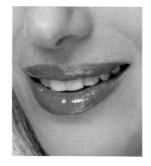

lip color is one of the quickest ways to set the mood of your overall look. You can go all out and define your lips with color, or you can use a clear gloss for a more natural look.

luminescence describes a foundation with light-reflecting qualities that creates a glowing, refined look. The light-reflecting properties contain specially shaped particles that bounce light away from imperfections, surface lines, and wrinkles, to create a more youthful appearance.

mascara is a product designed to coat each eyelash with color to give you full, long, thick, and dark lashes. Mascara makes your eyes stand out. There are many formulas, designed to give you a variety of effects.

matte is used to describe lipsticks, eyeshadows, foundations, powders, and blushes that have absolutely no shine and appear flat. Matte lipsticks tend to be drier than glossy or satin types, but they stay on longer. Matte foundations are excellent on shiny and oily skins and are best for imperfect complexions. There are also matte products, such as powders and crèmes, that help fight oils during the day.

melasma is also known as chloasma or the "mask of pregnancy." In this acquired condition, the skin on the face and neck slowly develops brown patches. Melasma usually occurs during the second or third trimester of pregnancy. It can also develop in women taking oral contraceptives or hormone replacement therapy or people who have had excessive sun exposure. The brown patches are attributed to an increased amount of pigment in the skin.

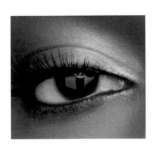

metallic describes lipsticks, eyeshadows, and eye pencils with a shiny, reflective metal finish. They are usually trendy and fun. They look fantastic on dark or ebony skin because they show up so well, but they can be too harsh for very pale or more mature skin.

mica is a small particle used in cosmetics; ground very finely, it produces shine and shimmer in a product. Most often used in eyeshadows, blushes, and lipsticks, mica can be colorless or a variety of shades.

midtone is a neutral, natural eye color that is swept across the eyelids to help define and shape the eyes. The midtone shade should be a natural extension of your complexion and is the second step in the three-color layering technique for the eyes. It is middle in depth in shade, darker than your highlight shade and lighter than your contour shade.

mousse is a texture that resembles that of a fluffy whipped dessert. It's most common in foundation and blush, making them lighter in weight and more sheer in coverage, which also tends to help them blend into the skin more completely.

mute or muting is to make a color appear less

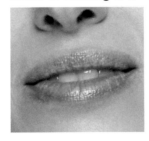

intense. For example, taking a bright pink and adding or layering another shade (possibly a beige) on top, to tone it down to a much softer and more natural pink.

noncomedogenic is a term used to describe a product that is formulated to not clog your pores, which helps prevent blackheads from forming.

oil absorbers are ingredients added to a formula that help absorb natural oils secreted by your skin throughout the day. Some foundations contain oil absorbers to prevent your face from becoming oily and help your foundation stay in place all day.

oil-free describes a product without added oils in its formula. This doesn't mean the product does not contain moisturizers; it simply means that the moisture does not come from added oils.

opaque is a finish that provides absolute coverage, allowing very little skin to show through.

pH level refers to the acidity or alkalinity of your skin. Your goal is to use products that maintain a neutral balance on your skin. You never want your pH level to be higher than 7, which is neutral—neither acidic nor alkaline—and is considered balanced. A high pH level (above 7, or alkaline) in your skin can cause the pigments in your cosmetics to change color once applied.

polymer is a small ingredient or particle that is added to a product, to help it cling to whatever it's applied to, adding bulk, volume, and length. It's most commonly used in mascara and is the ingredient that creates the longer, thicker appearance of your lashes.

porosity is the skin's ability to absorb and hold moisture. Moisturizer can "even out" the porosity of your skin and help your foundation, primer, or concealer go on more smoothly.

powder refers to talc-like products, such as eyeshadow, blush, and face powder. For example, face powder, which is used for setting foundation and concealer, gives your face a smooth finish and keeps shine under control. Powder comes in multiple forms, including loose and pressed.

primer is a product used underneath other products, to create a smoother finish. Makeup primers create a barrier between your skin and anything applied over the product. Some are designed to prevent products applied over them from seeping into fine lines and places they do not need to be. Primers also keep your makeup in place much longer, as you go through your day.

rosacea is a skin disorder that leads to redness and pimples on the nose, forehead, cheekbones, and chin. Rosacea can look a great deal like acne, but blackheads are never present.

satin refers to a formulation that's neither as flat as matte nor as shiny as shimmer. A "soft satin finish" is often used to describe foundations and liquid cosmetics that give a soft, smooth finish to the skin. Satin products have a sheen to them but are not shiny. Satin eyeshadows are particularly good for mature skin, because they glide on smoothly and add a soft sheen to the skin.

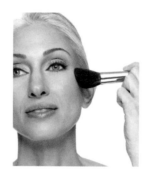

sculpting describes the process of reshaping a feature or even the face. In terms of makeup, it means using multiple depth levels of a product to visually reshape a feature's appearance; for example, sculpting a round (or full) face to look thinner or making a hooded eyelid look less full and fleshy. These effective techniques can make you look much more youthful.

sheer is a thinner, more transparent finish than matte or opaque and gives the skin a glow. It usually contains silicone, which allows makeup to glide on easily. The product clings less and covers more smoothly than an opaque product does. Sheer products seem to disappear into the skin, giving it a soft, more natural appearance. Sheer foundation is fabulous for mature women, because it helps their skin appear brighter and fresher, without drawing attention to fine lines.

silicone refers to any of a number of polymers containing alternate silicon and oxygen atoms that act in cosmetics as adhesives and lubricants, helping them adhere to the skin. This ingredient really helps a product become one with the skin. It can also make a product water-repellent.

skin tone describes your skin color, and it ranges from very dark brown to almost colorless (appearing pinkish-white due to the blood in the skin). Skin tone is determined by the amount (depth) and type (olive, yellow, pink, bronze, or ebony) of the pigment melanin in the skin.

stippling is a blending technique used for concealers and foundations or crème-type products. It's especially effective for blending out the edges of concealers. Stippling is also a great way to carefully apply one product over another. Just place some product, such as foundation, on your fingertips or a sponge and apply in a gentle patting motion, to avoid disturbing or erasing the product you've already applied underneath, such as concealer.

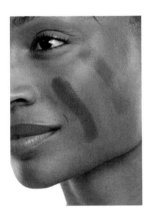

stripe test is a technique in which you apply multiple stripes of foundation to the skin, to test whether or not its color matches your skin color. You cannot get a perfect foundation match without conducting this test—it is a must.

t-zone describes the center of your face and includes the center of your forehead, nose, and chin. This area can have a slightly different texture than the rest of your face—larger pores, for example, which excrete more oils and give your skin a tendency to get shiny or oily more easily than the rest of the face.

texture is the consistency of a product—the feel or weight of the product on your skin. For example, a blush can have a creamy or a powdery feel to it. Foundation comes in many textures, including crème, powder, and liquid. Texture describes the form of a product but not the finish. Foundation can have a dewy, creamy, sheer, matte, or satin finish, while lipsticks can be glossy, matte, or sheer.

tinted describes a product that gives the skin the slightest hint of color. Pigments in these products are very light, to just slightly add color and give the sheerest coverage possible.

undertone is the underlying tone of a color. It's the base from which the color is formed. For example, your skin can have an olive undertone. A warm shadow or blush has a yellow undertone, while a cool color has a blue undertone.

vitiligo is a condition in which patches of skin lose their pigmentation because the pigment-producing cells, the melanocytes, are attacked and destroyed. It can affect the skin, mucous membranes, eyes, inner ear, and hair, leaving white patches. The most common type of vitiligo is vitiligo vulgaris. See also Hypopigmentation.

water-based describes the formulation of a product that can be removed with or is soluble in water. These formulas generally are considered to be less irritating to the skin than formulas that require special creams or other removers. This is the formulation most commonly used in foundation.

water-resistant describes a product that resists water. Although it will not smudge or smear when in contact with moisture or water, it cannot be submerged in water without running or being otherwise affected.

waterproof describes a product that repels water—it does not allow water to penetrate it. A waterproof product can be completely submerged in water and will not smear, smudge, or run.

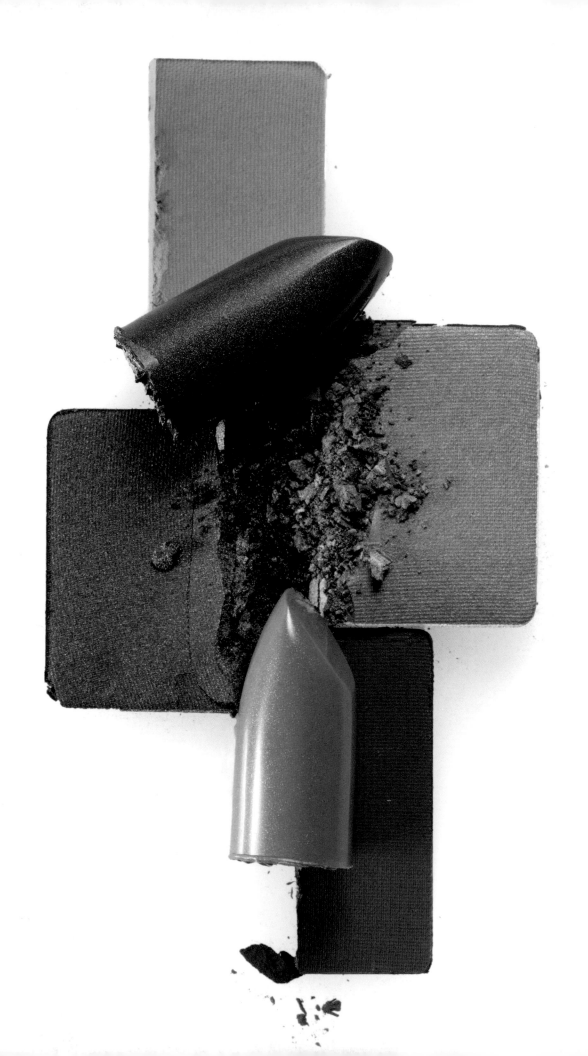

3

you need to know

One of the most confusing issues for a woman who wants to look younger by using makeup is figuring out which products to use. There are so many products available that it is easy to become confused and overwhelmed when trying to make the best choices. You simply do not know what will work for you. What formula of foundation will look the best? Which type of blush is the easiest to apply? Should you wear lip gloss?

If you go to a department store, you are often hit with an endless number of products that the salesperson just wants to sell to you. If you go to a drug store, there is no one there to help you. Which is better?

I think the absolute best thing you can do is educate yourself about all products, so you can make educated decisions about the products you want or need. The more you know about each product, the better able you are to make the right choices for yourself. In this chapter, we will discuss the choices available and help you learn which products will work the best for you and your needs.

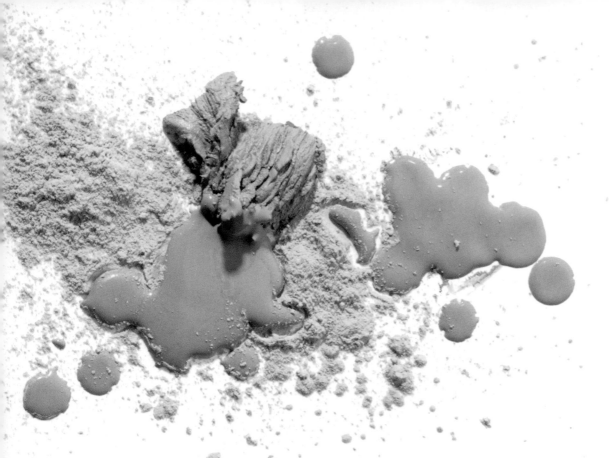

foundation

Foundation is the most important item of makeup you will ever purchase, and, while the right formula can literally erase years, the wrong formula can add years. Why is foundation so important? It can make your skin appear flawless and natural and give it a healthy glow. It can cover imperfections and blemishes and smooth out uneven skin tones, making your skin look more youthful. Wearing it correctly can do more for your appearance than almost any other makeup product. Unfortunately, foundation can also be one of the most difficult products to choose correctly. Using the right formula is so important, because the wrong one is almost guaranteed to make you look older.

When choosing foundation, there are two things to consider. The first is to match your skin tone and its depth level, so that your foundation looks natural. The second is to match your skin type with the correct foundation formula. For example, if your skin is oily, the oils from your skin can mix with the product and make your foundation appear blotchy and uneven. So you will need a foundation with oil absorbers in it. If your skin is dry, you will need a foundation with moisturizers in it, to help your skin look youthful and fresh. Wearing the correct foundation formula for your skin type can help your foundation stay on longer and your skin look younger.

My professional advice? Treat yourself to the best foundation you can afford. Higher-priced foundations usually contain higher-quality pigments, which last longer on your skin and give a more flattering appearance than less-expensive brands. They also usually contain higher-quality moisturizers and oil absorbers, which helps them perform better, as well. Cheaper foundations containing fewer and inferior pigments generally don't wear as long.

Your skin is the most important part of your makeup look, so making it appear its absolute youngest and freshest is also important. Foundation and powder are the bases of flawless-looking skin, so try to buy the best. If your skin looks flawless, I promise, you will look younger.

We now have a lot more to work with, when it comes to foundation formulations. Thanks to modern technology, many foundations can appear almost invisible. Foundations now contain all kinds of new light-reflecting ingredients that hide your flaws without having to pile on lots of product. You can choose from a variety of textures and formulas that will give you different types of coverage and finishes. A product's consistency and the way it goes onto the skin is the key to even, flawless coverage.

The goal is to look as if you're not wearing any foundation at all—you simply want to give the illusion of having healthy, young-looking skin. So, when it comes to choosing and using foundation, pay close attention to the changing texture of your skin, and change your foundation accordingly. Your skin changes as you age, and you must change your foundation to match, if you want to continue looking young.

liquid foundation is the most popular and is suited to most—if not all—skin types. It is available in every type of formula for every skin type, from oil-free, oil-absorbing formulas, which work best on oily skin, to moisturizing formulas, for dry skin. As many women age, their skin tends to become much drier, so they definitely need a formula with moisture in it. Liquid foundation gives varying degrees of sheer to medium coverage, depending on the brand and the formula, so you can choose the amount of coverage you want. When applied, it provides more coverage than a tinted moisturizer but less than a crème or stick foundation. You can purchase liquid foundation in a bottle or a tube.

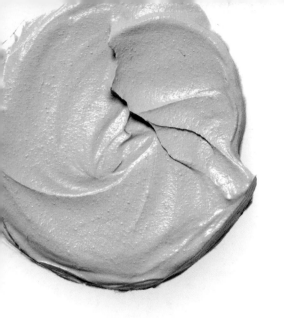

crème foundation is smooth and creamy and is formulated for normal to very dry complexions. One of the most moisturizing formulas you can use, it gives the skin a natural finish, while offering the most coverage. I find it very versatile, because, although it has a thicker and heavier consistency, you can make it more sheer simply by applying it with a damp sponge (which also allows you to control the coverage). Also, because of its great coverage, it can even be used as a concealer if you only have minor imperfections. Crème foundation is great for dry skin. However, if you have dry, flaky skin, beware, because it can look cakey, and the result can be slightly dull and heavy-looking.

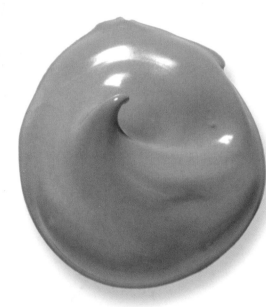

mousse foundation is actually crème foundation with a whipped consistency. This lightweight foundation provides even coverage and resists creping, so it's the perfect choice for aging skin. Formulated for normal to dry skin, mousse foundation generally comes in a jar, rather than a compact, and is generally lighter and more sheer than its compact counterpart. It evens out the skin tone without appearing heavy. I use mousse-textured formulas a lot, because they seem to sink into the skin rather than sit on top of it, giving great coverage that appears very natural. Unlike heavier crème formulas, they do not collect in fine lines and so are fabulous on mature skin. This is probably my favorite formula, due to its coverage, but it still looks natural, never heavy or thick.

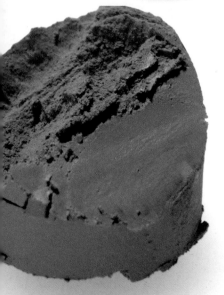

stick foundation is essentially a crème foundation and concealer in one neat package. Best for normal to dry skin, it is a good option for women who want more coverage. It offers maximum coverage for imperfections and ruddy and uneven skin tones. Stick foundation provides quick coverage, but it can look a little heavy on clear skin, which doesn't need a lot of coverage. The beauty of this formula is that you can simply dot it where you need it, rather than applying it to your entire face. Then you blend in powder and go.

crème-to-powder foundation is quick and simple. Formulated for normal to slightly oily skin, its creamy texture dries to a powder finish, so you don't need an additional dusting of powder to set it. This formula is kinder to oily skin than its crème counterparts, because the powder helps cut down on excess shine. A crème at heart, it provides more coverage than a liquid or tinted moisturizer but less coverage than its moisturizing crème counterparts (crème and stick).

tinted moisturizer is a moisturizer with a little added color. This formula works best on normal to dry skin and provides sheer, lightweight, breathable coverage with a fresh, nearly naked finish. The sheerest coverage of all the foundation formulas, it's perfect for use during the summer months, when you feel like wearing next to nothing on your skin. Tinted moisturizer evens out the skin tone while providing minimal coverage and, due to its sheerness, is the easiest to apply. Many brands contain sunscreen, which means one less step in the morning.

powder compact is a dual-finish powder foundation that provides quick, convenient, sheer-to-medium coverage and is packaged in a nice neat compact. It is formulated for normal to oily skin; on dry skin, it looks chalky. It goes on like a pressed powder but contains emollients and pigments that provide more coverage than a pressed powder. It's perfect for young women, because it is low in oils and moisturizers and doesn't clog pores, which helps cut the risk of breakouts. It provides all the coverage that most young women need and is easy for them to apply. Dual-finish powder has its place in the makeup bag of more mature women, too; it's a great choice for touch-ups when you're on the go and you want more coverage than a pressed powder. The tool you use to apply the powder determines the amount of coverage. Applied with a brush, it gives you sheer coverage. Applied with a sponge, it gives you more complete coverage.

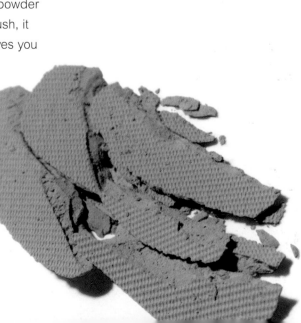

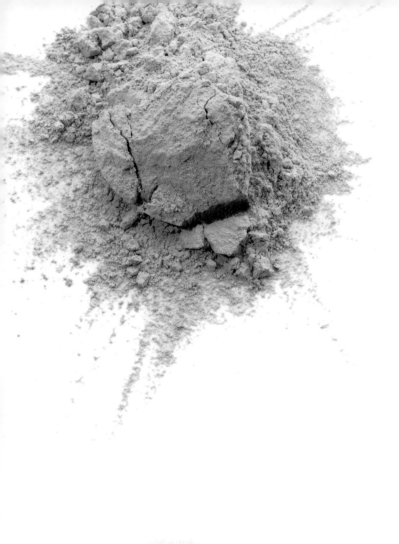

pigmented mineral powder is a loose powder that adheres to the skin, providing medium to full coverage. It is formulated for normal to oily skin; like dual-finish powder, it can appear chalky on dry skin. In addition to giving you coverage, it also contains vitamins and minerals, which make it great for sensitive skin. It works much like a dual-finish powder foundation and is simple to apply with a brush or a sponge. Applied with a brush, it gives you medium coverage. Applied with a sponge, it gives you full coverage. Regardless of which tool you choose, the more layers you apply, the more coverage you will get. Be careful, though: due to its powder consistency, too much of this formula can look cakey. Mineral powder generally does not contain preservatives, and, like tinted moisturizer, it often contains sunscreen.

aerosol spray foundation is foundation in an aerosol spray can. This formula provides maximum coverage with staying power. Most formulas work on all skin types and are water-resistant. Spray foundation was created to mimic what professional makeup artists call airbrushing (using a machine that sprays a fine mist of foundation). You simply spray it over your face, and it releases a mist of foundation, giving you complete coverage. After you spray it on, you can use a sponge or a brush to blend it in and help it look more natural. I find, however, that it looks heavier and less natural than other foundation options

tip:

Here's a *looking younger* secret: If your skin tends to flake, be sure you exfoliate to rid yourself of that top layer of dead, dry skin before applying a crème foundation.

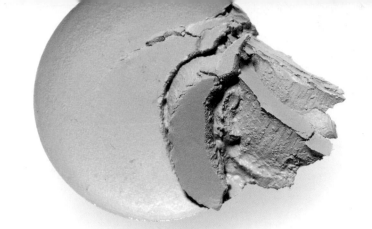

concealer

Concealer can be your best friend or your worst enemy, depending on which one you choose. Concealer comes in a multitude of formulations and textures, and because different textures are used for different problem areas, it's important to match it to the problem area. For example, a concealer used to cover under-eye areas should always be moist and creamy, whereas a concealer designed to cover breakouts or broken capillaries should be much drier in texture, so it will adhere better and last longer. If you use the wrong formula, your concealer can actually draw more attention to the problem you are trying to conceal.

stick concealers provide full coverage. They vary in dryness and texture—some are creamier, and some are much less moist. Stick concealers cover everything from dark circles to prominent blemishes and skin discoloration. When using this formula to minimize under-eye circles, be sure the texture and consistency is creamy enough to blend well and keep the area hydrated, so fine lines are not accentuated. Using a creamier texture helps keep the delicate skin under the eyes looking its most flawless. If you are covering other types of spots on your face, such as blemishes, dark spots, or veins, choose a stick that is a little drier in texture, so it will hold longer.

pot concealer provides similar coverage to stick (full), but it is formulated with more moisturizing ingredients and is not quite as thick. Perfect for concealing flaws, this is the form of concealer most commonly used by professionals because of its great coverage and versatility. As with stick concealers, there are many formulas out there, so find the one most suited to your needs. Although usually creamy, it is also available in drier, oil-free formulas that are used to cover discolorations such as blemishes and hyperpigmentation (because the drier it is, the better it will adhere).

tube concealer has a light, creamy texture that is less likely than other formulas to collect in fine lines, making it great for mature skin. It provides terrific coverage and is perfect for covering dark under-eye circles because it is moist and easy to blend. However, it does not have the staying power of drier formulas, so it might not be the best choice for other spots and discoloration on the face. Tube concealers can be mixed with moisturizer or foundation to create a sheerer product.

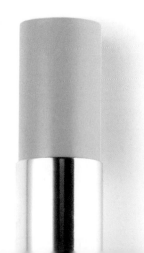

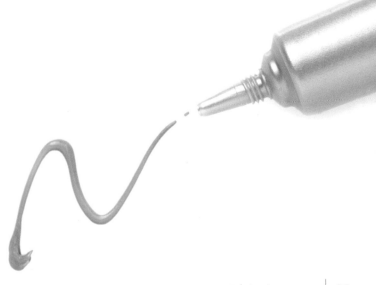

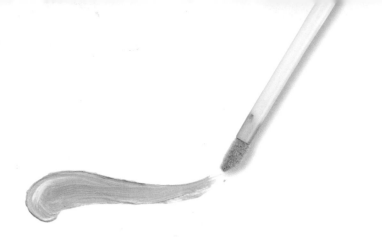
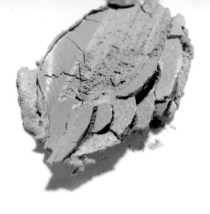

wand concealer provides the lightest and sheerest texture of all concealer formulas; it blends in easily and looks very natural, although it can settle into fine lines if not completely blended (due to the nature of the texture). If you use the proper shade, you can apply it without a foundation, because it blends so easily into bare skin. A wand concealer provides a quicker, slightly denser coverage than liquid foundation but less coverage than most other concealer formulas, and they are absolutely fabulous for a fast repair (because of their convenience). Some dry to a powder finish that is great for covering facial blemishes, because the powder clings, making it longer-wearing.

pencil concealers effectively cover tiny imperfections, such as broken capillaries, blemishes, veins, and any other tiny flaws. You simply draw it on (which is what makes it so amazing). Draw it all along a vein, or draw it right on a blemish or any other spots. With an exact color match, flaws can be concealed with exact precision and without a lot of blending. Pencil concealers are also terrific for fixing lip lines. Use it around the outer edge of your lips to erase your natural lip line (so that you can draw on your new one) or prevent lip color from bleeding. No other formula compares to the convenience of this product, which can be easily carried with you.

oil-free compact concealer formulations are best used on the face to hide pimples and spots. They generally offer a long-wearing, dry texture that will not irritate breakouts and will stay right where you put them. Because of their wearability, they are perfect for effectively covering blemishes, age spots, and hyperpigmentation (any type of spot on the face). But keep in mind that, because of their dry texture, they are the wrong choice for covering dark, under-eye circles—they will make the area appear dry and cakey.

highlighter pen is one of the most amazing makeup innovations of the past few decades. It contains light-reflecting particles, which bring forward recessed areas of the face and hide minor flaws. This is not a concealer—it is a highlighter (I stress this because many women are confused about the pen's use). It works by highlighting (bringing out) recessed areas, such as the dark shadows created by bags, wrinkles, deep creases, and the inside corners of your eyes, and making them look even with the rest of the face. Applying the highlighter to a shadowed area brightens it and makes it appear less distinct. There are many brands out there, and some can look dry (chalky or cakey), so be sure to choose one that looks fresh and natural.

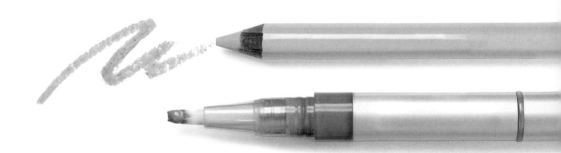

powder

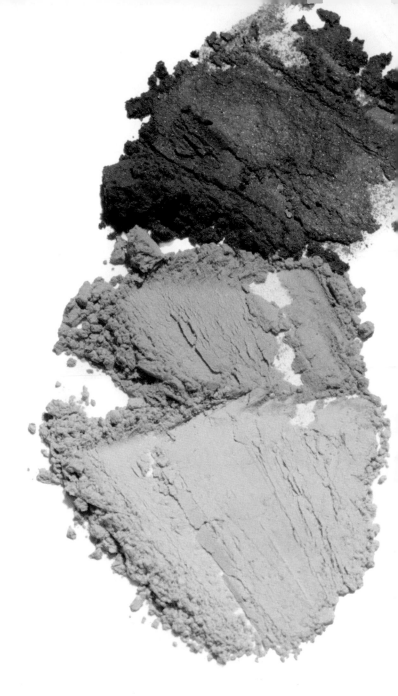

Many women think using powder will make them look older, but this is not true! Powder is your friend. A good, quality powder helps makeup look natural and, therefore, youthful. Powder is important for many reasons, but foremost is that it sets your make-up, which will not last the day without it. Also, if you do not powder, your color products will not go on evenly and smoothly; instead, they will "catch" on different areas of the skin and look blotchy. Powder is the finishing step that helps the skin appear smooth and natural. You can even brush it on over a clean, moisturized face for a fresh, no-makeup look.

Powder comes in two basic forms: loose and pressed. Both will set your makeup and absorb excess shine and oil. Loose powder is more oil-absorbing than pressed powder. I prefer to use loose powder when I am first setting foundation and concealer. It gives me a better finish and prevents the need for touchups longer. Pressed powder is wonderful, because it is easy to carry and is useful for touch ups as you go through your day. If you have oily skin, powder is your best friend, a must, because it prevents excess shine from the oils in your skin, which can draw attention to textural flaws.

An important characteristic to look for in a powder is that it must be finely milled. The finer a powder is milled, the higher its quality and the less likely it is to cake on the skin. Finely milled powders feel like velvet, whereas less finely milled powders feel gritty.

tip:

When buying powder, a good test is to touch it; it should feel soft and silky (like velvet), not gritty. Apply a little of it to the back of your hand (there is more texture to the skin there, so you will see if it catches in the lines). It should look sheer and natural. If it is too heavy (not milled finely enough), it can look dry and chalky.

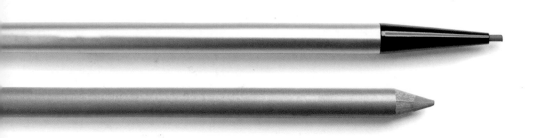

eyebrow color

I am often asked if every woman needs to fill in her brows. I would have to say no, *but* I find that approximately 95 percent of women do benefit from some brow color. You may not need a lot of filling in, but some will definitely help define and perfect your brow. Varying brow color types and formulas will give you varying results, from complete coverage to a soft, more natural effect. Choose the formula that helps you achieve your goal, whether it's slightly filling in or replacing what is just not there.

I will say it now, and I am sure that I will repeat it many times: Fuller brows make you look younger! So if you over-tweezed in your twenties, and the hairs never grew back, or they have just thinned with age, brow color is your best friend.

pencil is the most precise and probably the most common formula used to define the brows. Pencil provides great, full coverage and color when filling in your brows. It generally has a waxier consistency than other makeup pencils, which helps it last longer and adhere better to the brows. I find that slightly drier and harder formulas give the most natural application. Brow pencils come in two forms, mechanical and wood. A mechanical pencil (if it is a good one) will not need to be sharpened. Simply twist it to extend the product, then apply. If your pencil is wood, you control the point. Sharpen before each use, because the sharper the point, the better the application.

powder brow color is a matte, no-shimmer powder with a high pigment content. Powder provides the most natural look when filling in your eyebrows. It is all you need when you are just slightly filling in (when the shape of your brow is there, but it's sparse and you need to add a little bulk, because it will look completely natural, not like you just drew your brows on. It is usually applied with a narrow, stiff-angle eyebrow brush (turn to page 55 to find the perfect brush). It can be used to set brow crèmes and helps give pencils even more coverage and lasting power when you are creating a brow from nothing.

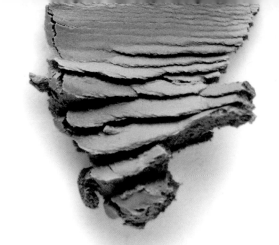

crème is the most dramatic-looking brow color, providing full coverage when filling in and defining your brows. A matte crème, is applied with a narrow, stiff, angled eyebrow brush and is best set with eyebrow powder, so it will last and not smudge. I find that it's the least natural-looking option. Even when set with eyebrow powder, it still can smudge (especially on oily skin). This is not the best choice for novices or for those who want a subtle look, because it is hard to make it look natural.

brow gel is like hair gel (or hair spray) for the brows. It's great for unruly eyebrows because it helps keep the brows in place. So, if your brows look out of place or lie less than perfectly, gel can keep them where you want them. Brow gels are available in tinted or clear formulas. Tinted formulas will not necessarily fill in your brows, but they do make the hairs you have look fuller and more noticeable (which might be all you want or need), while keeping everything in place. Clear formulas can help set the color (pencil or powder) already applied, while keeping your eyebrow hairs in place. I am not a big fan of the tinted versions, but I love the clear, which keeps brows looking perfect all day.

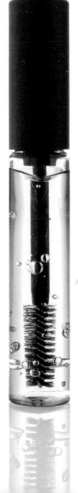

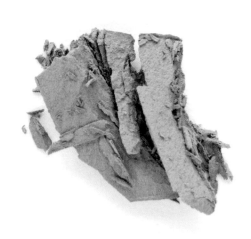

mascara

How can you live without mascara? You shouldn't. This is the most important element of your eye makeup, because of the definition it creates. Full, thick, dark lashes are a must if you want to look younger, because they help open up your eyes, which makes them look more alive and youthful.

I love mascara. It would be one of the first items I would take to a deserted island. I could not live without it. But enough about love! Mascara comes in multiple formulas that give you a variety of results. Of course, your application technique will also make a difference in your results (visit page 192 to get the scoop). Choose the formula that helps you achieve the look you want.

tip:

It's always better to apply two thin coats of mascara, rather than one thick, clumpy coat.

thickening mascara coats each individual lash from root to tip with particles that add bulk to the lashes and help them look thick and full. It is formulated with dark pigments, thick waxes, and silicone polymers, which create the density. This formula is the thickest of all formulas, because the goal is to increase lash size. Yes, sometimes size really does matter!

lengthening mascara contains plastic polymers that cling to the tips of the lashes, making them appear longer. Thinner than a thickening formula, it does not add bulk, just particles that attach to the end of your lashes and add precious length.

defining mascara coats each individual lash and keeps them separated and defined. If a mascara is labeled as defining, it usually means that it does not contain particles that add bulk and length to your lashes; it simply coats each lash with color, for subtle definition. Defining mascara usually appears the most natural.

waterproof mascara means that the formula has been shown not to smudge or smear when subjected to (submerged or totally dowsed in) water or tears in tests. Most mascaras are available in a waterproof formula. It's a harder to remove than other formulas, so be sure you use a good eye-makeup remover for cleansing.

water-resistant mascara resists smearing and smudging but is not fully waterproof. Look up water-resistant in the dictionary and you will see that the word is defined as resisting, though not entirely preventing the penetration of water, and that is the perfect description. It won't hold up to swimming or sweating, so it's not a good choice for a sports mascara.

curling mascara is supposed to help curl your lashes as you apply it. I am only listing it because it has been a big craze, but I have not found these mascaras to curl enough to provide the benefits you need. The theory behind them is that they contain polymers that contract (shrink) once applied, causing your lashes to curl and lift. Not my personal favorite!

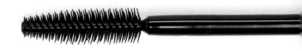

choosing a mascara wand

Most women do not realize that the bristles and shape of a mascara wand have just as much impact on the look of their lashes as the mascara's formula and their application technique. There are many wand options out there today, everything from a rubber brush to a comb. In the past, your wand choices were much less varied, making one easier to choose. Following are some key things to consider when deciding what you want and need from your brush or applicator. Keep in mind that, regardless of wand type, you still ultimately have control of your finished look, through the application technique you choose. Visit page 192 to learn the *looking younger* way to apply mascara.

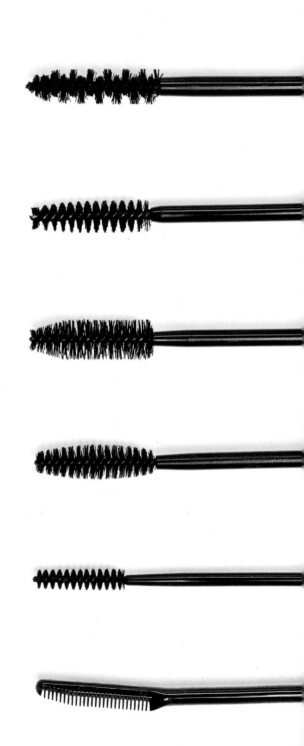

- A wand with long, fat, full, thick, dense bristles will help thicken and lengthen your lashes as you apply your mascara, because it coats each and every lash with product.

- A wand with short, dense bristles (it might even resemble a screw) helps define your lashes, because it allows you to coat each lash with a thin coat of product from the root to the tip.

- A wand with bristles that taper from short at the tip to longer in the middle or base (it might taper from thin to thick to thin, like a football), defines, thickens, and lengthens lashes. It enables you to perform detailed defining work with the tip (because the tip bristles are shorter), while giving you volume and length from the bristles in the middle and at the base of the brush (because the bristles are longer and fuller).

- A wand with widely spaced rubber bristles defines and separates your lashes, giving you a thin, even coating of product on every lash.

- A wand shaped like a comb defines and separates each and every lash. It provides a thin coat of product while combing and separating each lash, which completely eliminates clumping and prevents lashes from getting stuck together.

eyeliner

Eyeliner is definitely an option, not a must, when applying your makeup. There are definite benefits to wearing eyeliner, but only if you choose the right formula for your desired effect. Poorly applied eyeliner will make you look older and your eyes appear smaller, whereas properly applied eyeliner opens up the eyes for a more youthful look.

pencil is the most commonly used eyeliner, simply because it is the easiest to control, and if you make mistakes, they are easy to fix. There are many pencil textures available. Some are dry and hard, some are creamy and glide on effortlessly. In the past, many women felt the need to soften their hard, dry pencils with a lighter or a match. Thankfully, most pencils now contain silicone, which enables them to glide on smoothly and makes them easy to smudge and blend. The best choice is a pencil with just enough silicone to glide on easily, but not so much that it smears or travels. Be sure your pencil is at least water-resistant, so it will stay put and not smudge. Pencils come in mechanical and wood types. A mechanical pencil does not need to be sharpened; simply twist to extend the product, then apply. If your pencil is wood, you control the point; sharpen before each use, because the sharper the point, the better the application.

liquid eyeliner is a colored liquid that is applied with a fine-tip applicator for perfect precision. You will find multiple applicator options, depending on the brand and formula—everything from a fine-tipped brush (the most common) to a felt-tip pen or pointed, sponge-tip applicator. Liquid liner is usually long-wearing and looks the most dramatic. Because of this, it might not be the best choice if you want to create a soft definition along your top lash line. Liquid liner is a good choice to use with strip false eyelashes, because it can successfully conceal the band of the false lashes. Liquid eyeliner should only be applied along the top lash line, never along the bottom lash line, because it looks too harsh and unnatural.

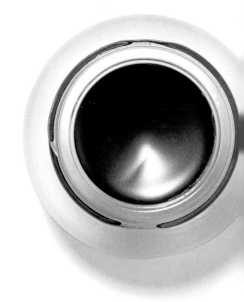

crème or gel eyeliners are usually packaged in a pot and are applied with a fine-tipped brush. They provide a similar effect to liquid eyeliner, which means they can be quite dramatic. Also, because they look much like liquid eyeliner, you should only apply them along the top lash line, never along the bottom lash line, where they will look harsh and unnatural. One big positive is the fact that they dry much quicker than liquid, which makes them easier to use without smearing the liner all over the place. They also tend to be long-wearing.

cake eyeliner is a pressed powder–like product that is usually applied with a damp eyeliner brush. It may look like an eyeshadow, but it is actually more heavily pigmented and denser in texture. Most formulas (the classic versions) work best when using a damp brush, but with some formulas, you can use your brush dry. Using a cake formula with a dry brush provides a subtle effect. When applied with a damp brush, it provides more dramatic definition. Dampened cake eyeliner gives a similar effect to liquid eyeliner, but it's much easier to control.

tip:

You can use any powder eyeshadow as eyeliner; all you need is the perfect brush (turn to page 57 to find the perfect brush) to create the effect you want to achieve. This will give you the absolute most natural and subtle definition along your lash line.

eyeshadow

Eyeshadow can do so much to bring attention to your eyes and wake up your face, making you look younger. If used correctly, it can reshape your lids and make them look their most beautiful. When choosing eyeshadow, you need to consider two things: the texture and the finish. Both make a big difference in the effect they create and how dramatic they look. And if your goal is to look younger, some choices are definitely better than others. Let's arm you with all the knowledge you need.

texture

powder shadows are available in loose and pressed forms. Both formulas vary in finish, from matte to shimmer and from iridescent to frosty. The pressed version is the most popular and the easiest to use, because it blends well without dripping too much color. Most makeup manufacturers offer the largest color choices in this texture. (Let's face it, it is the easiest to apply.) Loose powder eyeshadows work well and blend as well as their pressed counterparts, but you have to be a little more careful of shadow falloff. (This is no big deal: after dipping your applicator in shadow, just make sure to tap the excess off before you apply). They can be applied with a brush, sponge-tip applicator, or even your fingers, but I find that a brush gives you the best blend and results.

crème shadows are available in every finish; the most popular being mattes and shimmers. Most manufacturers carry a more limited shade selection of crème than powder eyeshadows. They are a great option if you have really dry eyelids, although be aware that many crème shadows can crease. Some crème eyeshadows dry to a powder finish, and they work the best. Many, if not most, are at least water-resistant; some are waterproof and long-wearing. For more intense color, you can apply a crème eyeshadow first, then follow it with a powder eyeshadow. But this will make the shadows harder to blend, so if you try this technique, be sure to place the color where you want it when you first apply it.

pencil shadows are eyeshadows in a convenient pencil form. They are useful for using around the eye close to the lash line, because they are sharpened to a point and can be applied with such precision. But they also work well anywhere on the eyelid. Their precision makes it easy to get the product right where you want and need it (whether it be lash line, crease, or brow bone). After application, you can simply smudge the line with your finger, a sponge-tip applicator, or a brush to blend and create the effect you want.

liquid shadows usually come in a shiny, metallic finish and are actually the hardest to use. Because liquid shadow doesn't blend easily, you must be very precise (be sure you get it right where you want it from the start), so it's best when applied with a brush. Liquid shadow is usually used either as an eyeliner or applied close to the lash line for color intensity.

finish

matte finish eyeshadow has absolutely no shine or shimmer and is the best for creating a natural, no-makeup look. It is also the best finish for midtone shades, which need to look very natural. Matte eyeshadows usually contain a higher level of pigment and work really well for reshaping and defining the eye. A matte shadow will draw absolutely no attention to any fine lines or crepe-like texture on your eyelids, so it's the perfect choice for helping you look younger.

shimmer shadows have a subtle sheen and give a hint of sparkle. Shimmer shadows offer sheer coverage, so that when you sweep on the color, you can still see the skin underneath. They generally contain multiple shades of mica (the shiny particles), which are actually sheer and see-through, softening their appearance on the skin. They typically won't collect in fine lines, which makes them a great choice for mature skin or when you want something more fun than matte. Light shimmer shadows work well for highlighting and bringing out recessed areas of the eyelid. Dark shimmer shadows add drama without being as harsh and intense as matte shades, because the shimmer particles reflect light and soften the final effect.

satin shadows fall perfectly between matte and shimmer. They are shinier than a matte, but not nearly as sparkly as a shimmer, so they give the eyelid a sheen without appearing sparkly or glittery. They are great for dry lids and create a natural look without the ashy effect that can result from a matte shadow. A satin finish is easy to wear and works well on all skin types, including mature skin.

frosted shadows provide the most shine or sheen. They can actually look reflective. A frosted eyeshadow gives you coverage that is more opaque than a shimmer shadow, covering the skin underneath it. The mica in a frost is usually one shade, most often a silvery white, and each little fleck of mica is opaque, as well. Because of this, they create the most drama and change in color when used, but the mica can collect in fine lines and draw more attention to them, so a frosted shadow is not the best choice for mature eyelids with fine lines, wrinkles, or a crepe-like texture. They usually come in fun, light pastel shades that look great on younger skin.

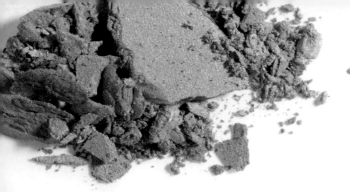

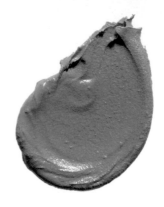

blush

Blush can be one of your best allies in the quest to look younger, by bringing an amazing youthful flush and glow to your cheeks. However, the formula, texture, and finish can make the biggest difference in determining whether your blush is your friend or your enemy. Most blush textures come in various finishes, such as matte and shimmer. Some formulas are easier than others to apply and use, while some have greater staying power. Different formulas also can give you differing degrees of coverage; some are sheer, and some contain heavier pigments, which provide more coverage and color intensity.

powder blush is pigment in a powder base. It's the most popular type of blush, because it's the easiest to control and use, and therefore it's usually available in the widest range of shades. Applied with a soft blush brush, it gives a dusting of color that works well with the majority of skin types. Powder blush is perfect for combination and normal skin and is the best choice for oily skin. If your skin is really dry, however, this formula might not be your best friend. Usually packaged in a pressed form (the most convenient and easy to carry), it can also be found in a loose version. Some formulas are matte, while some contain shimmer. The matte version tends to look the most natural and does not accentuate textural flaws in the skin.

crème blush is pigment set in a crème base. Its fresh, dewy finish gives the face a luminous, natural glow. A great choice for normal to dry skin, it's an especially good choice for dry skin, because it slides easily over the surface and blends into the skin. It works best when applied after your foundation and

before your powder so that it blends in more easily. Crème blush is not a good choice for oily skin, because it will not wear well. It also does not work well on skin with large pores, because it tends to accentuate them. It's great for those who do not need or want to wear foundation. Just apply it with your fingers or a sponge and work it into your skin.

gel blush is made up of pigment wrapped within silicone particles. It works best for women with normal to dry skin, because it won't last on oily skin. It smoothes nicely over bare skin to create a pretty, sheer, translucent glow. That's not to say you can't use it with foundation—you can. Just be sure to apply it before you powder. Gel blush is long-lasting, looks natural, and is easy to use. You can use your fingers or a sponge to apply it, then smooth it into the skin.

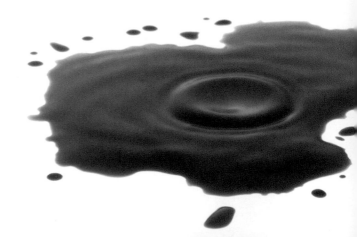

liquid blush or tint is actually a liquid that temporarily stains the skin. It works on all skin types. It is applied in a similar manner as the gel blush, but is a little more difficult to work with because it must be blended quickly, due to its staining quality. (Practice makes perfect!) It's waterproof, so you can expect it to last all day. Use either a sponge or your fingers to apply and blend it into your skin.

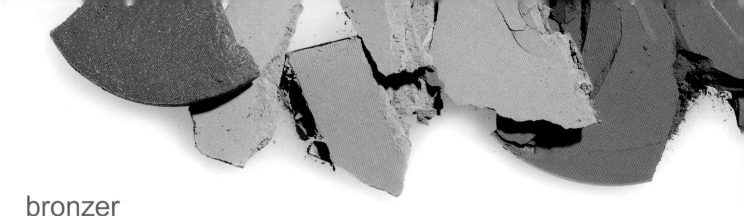

bronzer

Bronzer is the secret to having an eternally youthful glow. As you will soon discover, I think that every woman can benefit from bronzer. I honestly do not think I have ever applied makeup to anyone's face and not used bronzer. For me, going without bronzer is like running around naked. It finishes the face and takes off years. Bronzers are also available in many textures and finishes, and, once again (you are probably sick of hearing me say this!), choosing the right formula is the key to a youthful look.

powder bronzer, like powder blush, is the most popular type of bronzer, because it is so easy to control and blend. It is packaged in a variety of ways: pressed into a compact, loose in a tub, or even pressed into small balls or beads in a jar. Powder bronzer works for most skin types (normal, combination, and oily), but isn't the best choice for very dry skin. Powder bronzer finishes range from matte to a heavy dose of shimmer. I almost always choose a matte finish (except on really dark skin tones), because I think it looks the most natural. Also, because bronzer is used on such a large area of the face, too much shimmer can draw attention to the skin's textural flaws. Swept across strategic areas of the face with a brush, it can bring the skin to life.

crème bronzer is available in stick form or even in compacts. This formula works best on normal to dry skin, especially dry. It's perfect for days when you don't want to wear foundation but want that little extra glow, because it blends beautifully into bare skin. It can be applied with your fingers or a sponge.

gel bronzer works best on normal to dry skin and provides a much sheerer wash of color than other bronzers. Basically a sheer gel containing pigments, it is very easy to blend into the skin and works particularly well if you are trying to cover a large area of skin (legs, arms, body). This formula is most often packaged in a tube.

"bronzer is the secret to having an eternally youthful glow"

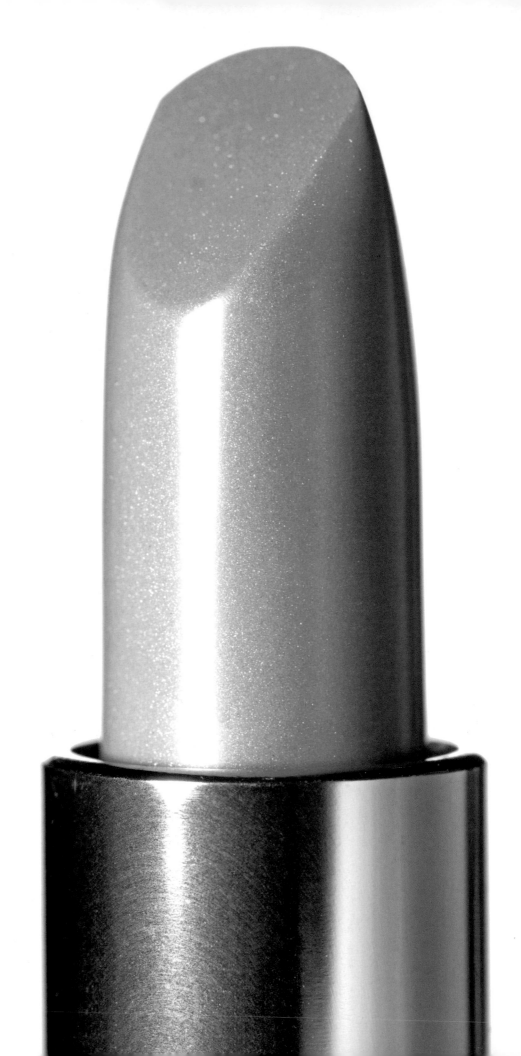

lip color

I think that, for most women, lip color is a very personal thing. One formula definitely does not work for everyone! Some women want a lot of coverage and moisture from their lipstick and/or gloss, while others prefer a sheer wash of color that looks and feels like it isn't even there. You will find numerous textures of lipstick and lip glosses out there, in a variety of finishes. Play, test, and try, until you find what you want in a lipstick or lip gloss. Keep in mind that moisture is always good for your lips; it helps them stay full and supple-looking, which, of course, makes them look younger.

matte lipstick delivers sophisticated, intense, full-coverage color with absolutely no shine. Because of its formulation, it stays on longer than other lipsticks, but it can be drying and may give your lips the feel and appearance of being dehydrated. Thanks to up-to-date technology, there are now some matte formulas that are not quite so dry and dehydrating, but they will not wear as long as the drier versions. Matte lipsticks are great in dark, intense shades, because they stay put and don't smear easily. You can always make a matte lipstick appear more luscious by applying a lip gloss on top.

crème lipstick contains more emollients than matte lipstick and provides a full coverage of moist (though not shiny) color. Most cosmetic lines offer the largest selection in this formula, because it is the most versatile and popular. It wears quite well, without being as dehydrating as matte lipstick. Keep in mind that there will still be different degrees of moisture in crème lipsticks, depending on the formulation and the brand. Crème formulas can have a natural, frosted, or shimmer finish.

sheer or **glaze** lipsticks provide a glossy, sheer wash of see-through color that allows your natural lip color to show through. These formulas contain pigments wrapped in a transparent hydrating gel. The coverage lasts longer than a gloss but not as long as a crème lipstick. It's terrific for a quick fix because, due to its sheerness, it doesn't have to be applied with precision.

long-wearing lipstick is a heavily pigmented formula with a very dry texture, which helps it stay put. It actually almost stains the lips, which gives them full coverage and is part of the reason it lasts so long. Long-wearing lipstick is extremely drying and dehydrating—definitely not your best choice if you are trying to look younger! I personally hate these formulas, because they tend to make your lips look smaller and shriveled. Luscious, full lips are always more beautiful, and this formula will not make that happen.

frost is a finish that provides a pale, shiny, metallic appearance to a lipstick. The metallic appearance is created by incorporating small flecks of a shine-producing material, which is solid and very reflective, into the lipstick formula. Lipsticks with a frosted finish generally provide opaque coverage and can make the lips appear a bit dry, so I don't recommend them if you are trying to give your lips a luscious youthful pout! They *are* good when used for layering over a satin-finish lipstick to lighten the depth of the shade.

shimmer is a finish that provides a beautiful, lustrous, glowing appearance to a lipstick. Like a frost finish, it is created by mixing into the formula tiny particles that produce shine. The difference between frost and shimmer is that the particles used in a shimmer finish are not opaque but sheer, so they create a glow without being extremely reflective. Shimmer lipsticks provide a nice, easy-to-wear, medium amount of coverage and can actually make lips look fuller (great for looking younger).

"glossy lips are always youthful and sexy"

gloss adds extreme shine and moisture to your lips. I *love* lip gloss, mainly because it immediately adds fullness and makes your lips look younger and kissable. It delivers a sheer to medium coverage layer of color to your lips. The only problem is that it does not have a very long wear life, so it needs frequent reapplication. Used correctly, it can make the lips look fuller and sexier and gives a fresh-and-alive look that's perfect for all age groups. You'll find it packaged in a wand, tube, or pot. Some formulas give more coverage than others, which means they will wear a little longer, so research (test drive) a few to find the formula or brand that gives you what you need. Check the label for key words that give you a clue to the wear time; "luster," "lacquer," "gel," "plastic," or "glass" can mean longer wear life, while "crystal," "wet," "transparent," "glaze," or "juicy" suggest a really high shine factor but probably a shorter wear time. Play away!

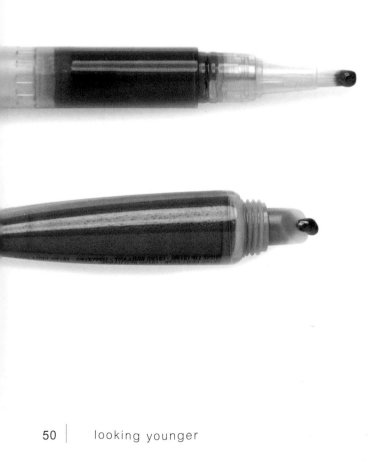

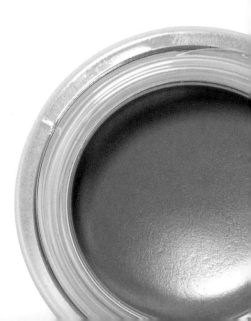

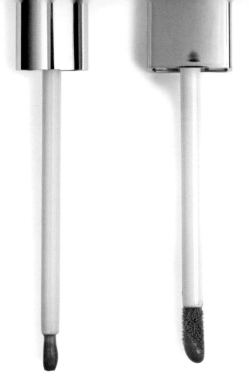

tip:

When you have finished applying lip liner, it should look invisible. Always blend your lip liner after application and before you apply your lip color.

lip liner is a pencil that helps define and reshape your lips. It can correct your lips' shape and prevents lip color from bleeding into fine lines. It can also be used over the entire lip, then topped with a lipstick or lip gloss. Using a lip liner greatly improves the staying power of any lip color. Lip liner pencil comes in two forms, mechanical and wood. A mechanical pencil does not need to be sharpened; simply twist to extend the product, then apply. If your pencil is wood, you control the point; sharpen before each use, because the sharper the point, the better the application.

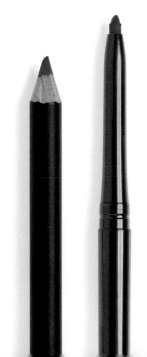

essential tools

As with anything you do in life, having at hand what you need to complete the task is imperative if you want to do a good job. When it comes to applying makeup, using the right tools will make your job much easier. Certain tools will give you the ability to apply any kind of makeup with precision and perfection.

For example, if you need to apply an eyeshadow to a specific area, using a brush designed specifically for that job allows you to get the powder right where you want it. Certain brush shapes allow you to create specific effects. Some sponges are better than others, due to their consistency and shape.

In this section, I'll take you through a variety of makeup tools; I'll tell you what they do, what makes some better than others, what to look for when buying them, and how to use them. For all the tools in this chapter, visit www.robertjonesbeauty.com to get what you need.

brushes

There are so many shapes, sizes, and types of brushes out there that choosing the right one can be very confusing. When it comes to brushes, though, price does make a difference: better brushes are more expensive. Also, I find that makeup artists' lines often offer better-designed brushes and more shape options, so you're certain to get the shape you need to get the job done correctly. Believe it or not, the shape of the brush head makes a huge difference in the effect it creates.

Here are some key points to consider when choosing your brushes.

the bristle: There are many different types of bristles, from natural, animal hair bristles to synthetic, and each can make a difference in your application. I've listed them here, in descending order of quality.

- **squirrel:** the most expensive and best bristle available. A natural bristle, it provides an even, smooth application and has the softest feel of all the bristle choices. It is used for powder product application, not crème. Because of the quality, a brush made of squirrel is expensive, but it's worth the investment.

- **pony:** a bristle that is one step below squirrel in quality. Powder and blush brushes are often made from this hair, but it is also used in other brushes. A natural bristle, it's best used for the application of powder products dry. Although the name might not suggest it, this bristle feels quite soft.

- **sable:** a high-quality bristle, commonly used for eyeshadow brushes. You will find more brushes made from this bristle than probably any other. This is also a natural bristle (made from the hair of a weasel-like animal called sable), so it provides an even, blended application. It is most commonly used for the application of powder products dry but can be used wet or damp for application of crèmes, such as crème eyeliner, crème eyeshadows, and applying eyeshadows damp. Although it can be used damp, never use a sable brush for applying foundation. The natural bristle will absorb all of the liquid from your foundation.

- **black silk:** the next level down in quality. This does not mean it isn't a great bristle, because some brushes provide better application when made of this hair. Also a natural bristle, it is actually a type of goat hair that has been treated to make it feel softer and smoother in its application. Best when used dry with powder products.

- **goat:** the least expensive natural bristle. Commonly used for blush and bronzer brushes, it is more cost-effective than squirrel, pony, or sable hairs. Sable hairs are too short to be used for longer-bristled brushes—blush, powder, and bronzer brushes, for example—so goat is often used instead. Like other natural-bristle brushes, it's used for applying powder products dry.

- **synthetic:** a bristle that is used for all liquid products. It is the bristle you want when applying liquids and crèmes, because it does not absorb moisture or liquid. It can be used to apply powder products, as well. This is the best bristle choice for foundation, concealer, and many eyeliner brushes, because of its compatibility with crèmes and liquids and its ability to be used damp. It is also very easy to clean, another reason it is perfect for foundation and concealer brushes.

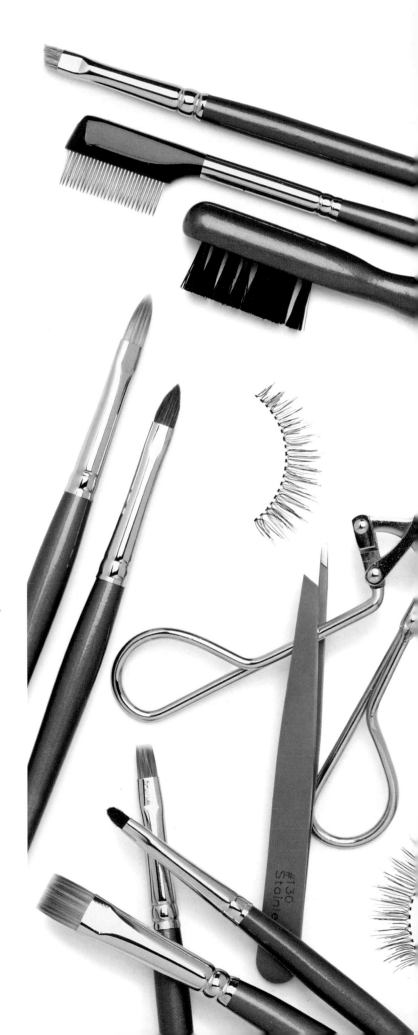

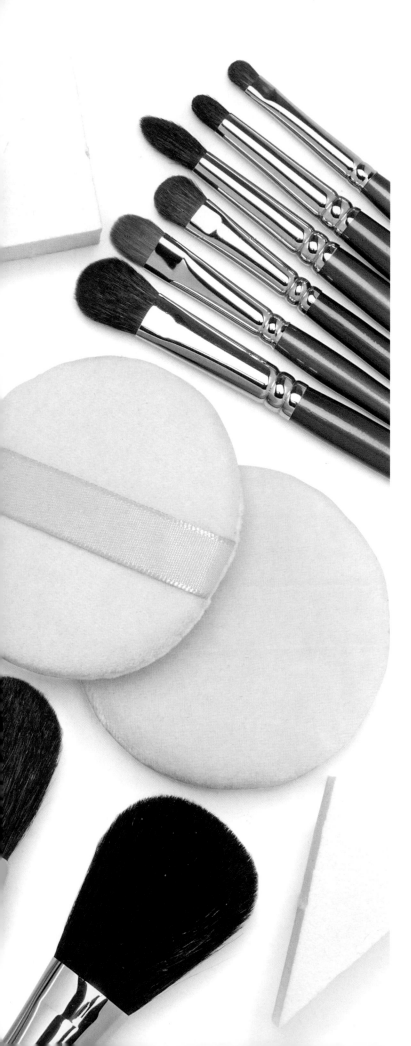

the handle: Be sure to choose a handle shape that feels comfortable in your hand. A comfortable handle makes a brush much easier to use. I prefer shorter handles—long handles never pack easily and can make the brush feel off-balance in your hand. The extra length, I find, gets in the way, but test the feel of a brush in your hand and choose the one that works best for you.

the head shape: The contour and shape of the brush head has a big impact on how well it applies a product. The length, the tapering of the hairs, the density, the quality, and the stiffness are all characteristics that make a huge difference in application. Blush and bronzer brushes need to be dense and full for more color deposit and a soft blended application, while an eyebrow brush needs stiff, compact bristles, for precise placement of color. Blending brushes should be very soft, so they don't irritate the skin when blending eyeshadow, while concealer brushes need to come to a bit of a point, for exact application. Eyeshadow brushes should be tapered, so they do not create hard lines; the ends of eyeliner brushes are usually flat and blunt, to create an exact line. So, shape does matter.

get the shape you need

This collection of brushes provides everything you need for every makeup application. I've used brushes from my own signature collection of make-up tools (www.robertjonesbeauty.com), so you can see my favorites.

eyebrow/eyelash brushes

- **angled eyebrow brush #1:** This is the perfect brush for applying color and shaping your brows. Its short, stiff bristles and narrow angle provide an exact application. The firmness of this brush is important to its ability to give precise placement of color. The edges of the brush are tapered, for softness of color application and to help in blending. It's traditionally used for applying brow powder and crème brow color, but is also your best friend for blending eyebrow pencil once applied.

- **brow brush:** It may look like a toothbrush, but it's not. This brush is the best for grooming and shaping your brows. It is the perfect shape for assisting in trimming your brows, because of its ability to brush the entire brow. It's also great for blending everything after all color applications.

- **eyelash comb #3:** An eyelash comb is a must for perfect lashes. After applying mascara, combing your lashes will help separate them and remove any clumps. Choose a comb with fine metal teeth, which provide the precision and separation that you can't get with its plastic counterpart.

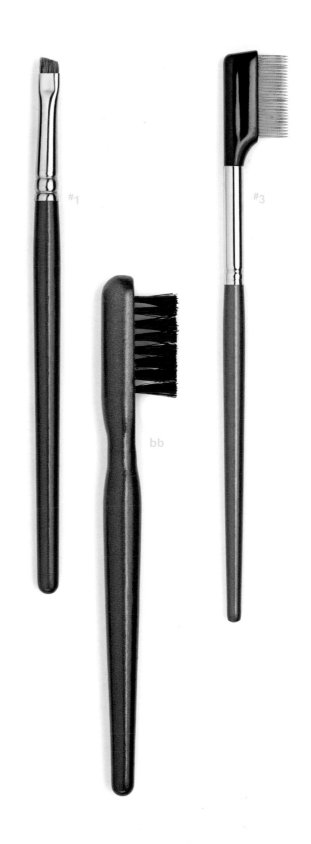

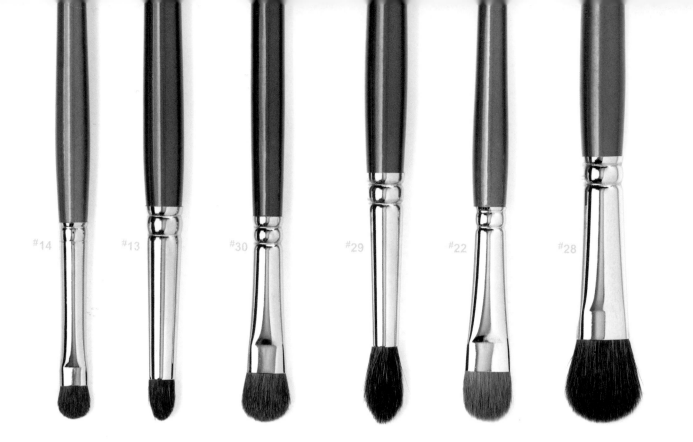

eyeshadow brushes

- **eyeshadow brush #14:** This sable brush is perfect for applying your highlight shade at the inside corner of the eye and the lower lash line (which you will discover opens the eyes for a wide-eyed, youthful look). It's also perfect for smudging liner and detailed color application.

- **eyeshadow brush #13:** This is a miracle brush no woman should be without. This precision-shaped squirrel-bristle brush is perfect for applying your favorite shade of eyeshadow along the lower lash line while giving you a smudged and blended effect (no harsh lines). Also perfect for creating a very defined line of color in the crease of the eye.

- **eyeshadow brush #30:** This precision brush, made of pony hair with the edges tapered for blending, is perfect for applying your most intense shade of eyeshadow along the lash line and into the outer corner of the crease of the eye. Its shape is ideal for creating a wide variety of looks and effects.

- **eyeshadow brush #29:** This tapered squirrel-bristle brush expertly applies your favorite mid-tone shade in the crease with precision, from the outer corner of the eye to the inside corner. The shape helps apply your color right where you want it and helps blend it to perfection.

- **eyeshadow brush #22:** Use this sable eyeshadow brush to precisely apply your highlight shade to your browbone and lid. It also works well for applying color anywhere to your eye when you want a brush with a slightly stiffer feel.

- **eyeshadow brush #28:** This soft squirrel brush is the perfect blending brush. It is a must when you're wearing more than one eye color. Keep this brush free of color, so you can use it to blend multiple shades of eyeshadow flawlessly. Use it over and across the lid after you have applied all your eyeshadow to blend all your shades together, without making the colors on your lid look muddy.

eyeliner brushes

- **eyeliner brush #41:** A tiny brush with big results, it's my secret weapon for eyes that grab attention with subtle perfection. Use this synthetic bristle brush to push color into your lash line; your eye color will really pop and your lashes will look absolutely thick. It's also perfect for very detailed lining.

- **eyeliner brush #18:** Use this wide, flat squirrel brush to precisely apply a line of bold or soft eye color along the lash line and to blend it up onto the lid. The shape of the brush makes your application the ultimate in ease—simply lay the brush flat on lid along your lash line and brush up. Great for helping you create a smoky eye.

- **eyeliner brush #40:** This flat, synthetic brush is used to line and define eyes with eyeshadow or to apply powder over your pencil liner to create a more subtle effect. It is also great for blending your pencil without adding color: Simply brush across the pencil to smooth and perfect the line. Perfect for wet or dry use, and works perfect for crème and gel eyeliner.

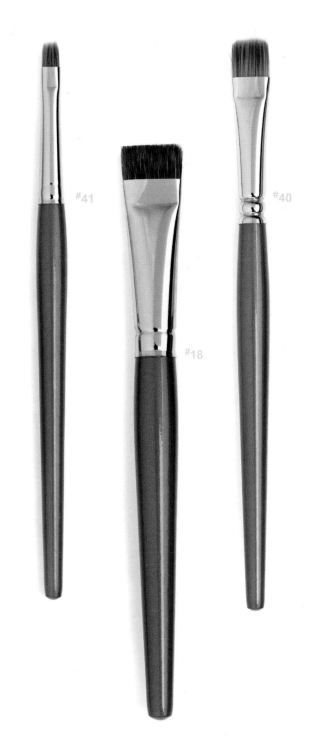

"making the perfect brush choices makes perfect application easier to achieve"

complexion and face-perfecting brushes

- **foundation brush #51:** Use this perfectly tapered, synthetic-bristle brush to apply cream or liquid foundation evenly and flawlessly onto the skin. It gives a smooth, even application, producing a flawless, perfect finish to your skin. The best tool for end-of-the-day foundation touch-ups, when you need to touch up your makeup to look your most beautiful but do not want to start your makeup application over from scratch.

- **blush brush #64:** The perfect apple-popping blush brush, made from the softest, highest-quality squirrel bristles. The round, full, tapered shape is perfect for applying color to the apples of the cheek, without leaving any harsh edges.

- **blush brush #62:** This is the ultimate blush and bronzer brush. Made with the softest squirrel bristles, it is the absolute best tool for applying blush or bronzer. Its full, round shape and expert tapering blend your blush or bronzer for the most professional application.

- **detailed powder/blush brush #73:** So many uses, so little time. This squirrel-bristle brush is so versatile, it's irreplaceable! It's the perfect tool for applying loose and pressed powder, unbelievable for removing excess loose powder after powder puff application, and priceless for detailed blush and face contour application. Its size and shape allow you to apply blush and bronzer with more exact precision.

- **jumbo powder brush #70:** A big, fluffy, black silk brush with a slightly tapered head shape that is perfect for brushing on loose powder smoothly, giving you sheer, even application. The black silk bristles increase the softness and quality of application.

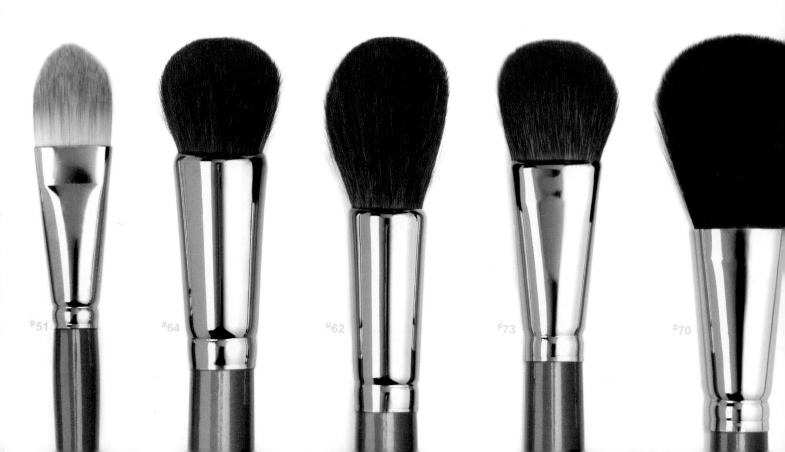

#51 #64 #62 #73 #70

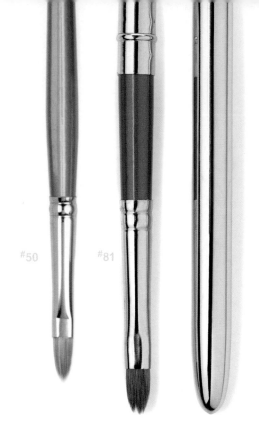

#50 #81

- **concealer brush #50:** This synthetic brush applies concealer with exact precision. Its tapered shape allows you to cover spots or flawed areas of the face without over-blending or overworking your concealer. Without this brush, you cannot cover the tiny flaw you want to disappear. A concealer brush is an absolute must-have.

- **lip brush #81:** This soft sable lip brush with a fine, tapered point applies lipstick and lip gloss with precision. The pull-apart top is great for travel or your purse, making it convenient for touchups anytime.

important brush fact

To get the best application and clarity of color, you need to clean your brushes regularly. The cleaner the tool, the better the application. You have a couple of cleansing options.

- The first is the simplest—professional brush cleansers. These can work beautifully. One great benefit is that most of them dry quickly, which makes them convenient. You dip your brush in the cleanser and wipe it off on a towel, cleaned to perfection.

- Your second option is to shampoo your brushes. Because brushes are made from hair, shampoo works great; the brushes will just take longer to dry. Dampen your brush, then, with a bit of shampoo in the palm of your hand, work the brush into the shampoo (a gentle baby shampoo works best and is not too harsh), and rinse. I find it best to lightly condition the brushes after washing (a light leave-in hair conditioner works well, because it is lightweight, but be sure to rinse it out afterwards), then rinse them. Finally, squeeze out the excess moisture (making sure to reshape the brushes, so that they dry to the correct shape) and lay them flat on a towel to dry.

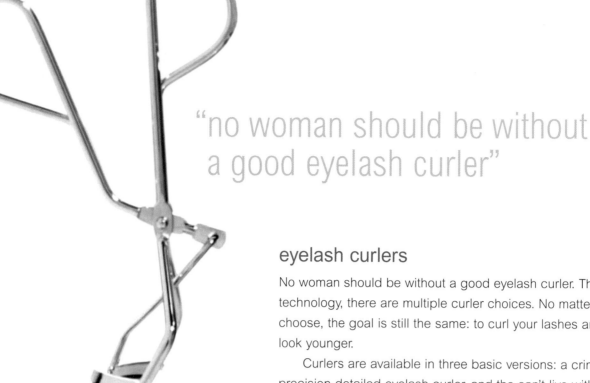

"no woman should be without a good eyelash curler"

eyelash curlers

No woman should be without a good eyelash curler. Thanks to modern technology, there are multiple curler choices. No matter which you choose, the goal is still the same: to curl your lashes and make yourself look younger.

Curlers are available in three basic versions: a crimp curler, a precision-detailed eyelash curler, and the can't-live-without-it heated eyelash curler.

- **crimp curler:** Usually metal, this is the most common and widely used curler and should only be used before applying mascara, never after. Be sure that the rubber pad or pads have curved edges to create a better curl, not a crimp. You must also be sure to replace your curler at least once a year, and replace the rubber piece at least once every six months. Turn to page 190 to learn proper curling technique.

- **precision-detailed curler:** This curler works just like a crimp curler, but its width makes it easier to get right to the lash root. I love it, because I can use it to curl the far inside and outside corner lashes that most crimp curlers miss. It is also easier to use on extremely short lashes.

- **heated curler:** This miracle product is a must-have! The beauty of this curler is that it works *after* you apply your mascara. (I am sure many of you have experienced the problem of having your mascara uncurl the lashes you have just curled.) Using a crimp or precision-detailed curler after applying mascara can rip lashes out. The heated curler actually uses the mascara as a curling catalyst, which helps the curl last all day. This curler will curl even the most stubborn lashes. Visit page 90 for usage instructions.

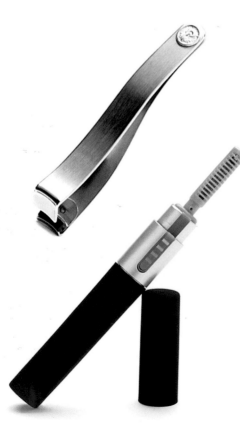

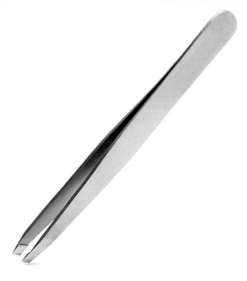

tweezers

Using a pair of quality tweezers is the only way to shape your brows perfectly. The best shape for the tweezers tip is slanted; if they are too pointed, you can injure yourself. The slanted tip allows you to be as detailed as you need and to get every little hair, without the danger of injury. Good-quality tweezers can be sharpened when they become dull and no longer grab the smallest hairs. (Manufacturers of good tweezers usually provide an address in the packaging, so you'll know where to send them for sharpening.)

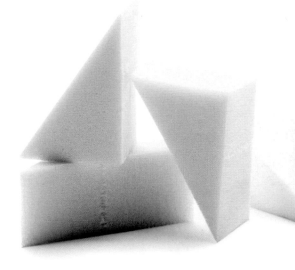

sponges

There are a couple of things to consider when choosing a sponge. First, look at the texture and quality. The better the sponge quality, the better-looking the application. So, price can definitely matter. The shape can affect how a sponge performs, as well. Depending on what you are using it for, the correct shape of sponge can make it easier to get makeup where you want it. The material from which it's made also has an impact on the application of product.

In today's world of beauty, you have many choices: your traditional triangular wedge, oval, and round sponges. One of my latest favorite tools is a new egg-shaped sponge, called the Beauty Blender. What makes it so amazing is the texture and shape, which allows you to create an airbrushed finish with your foundation. Also, it is latex-free, so it is a great option if you are allergic to latex.

powder puff

The best puffs are usually fluffy, with a soft velour texture. It's a good idea to invest in a quality powder puff, so you can launder it to keep it clean. Use it for applying pressed or loose powder. The beauty of a puff is that it allows you to really push the powder into the skin, creating a smooth, evenly applied, flawless finish.

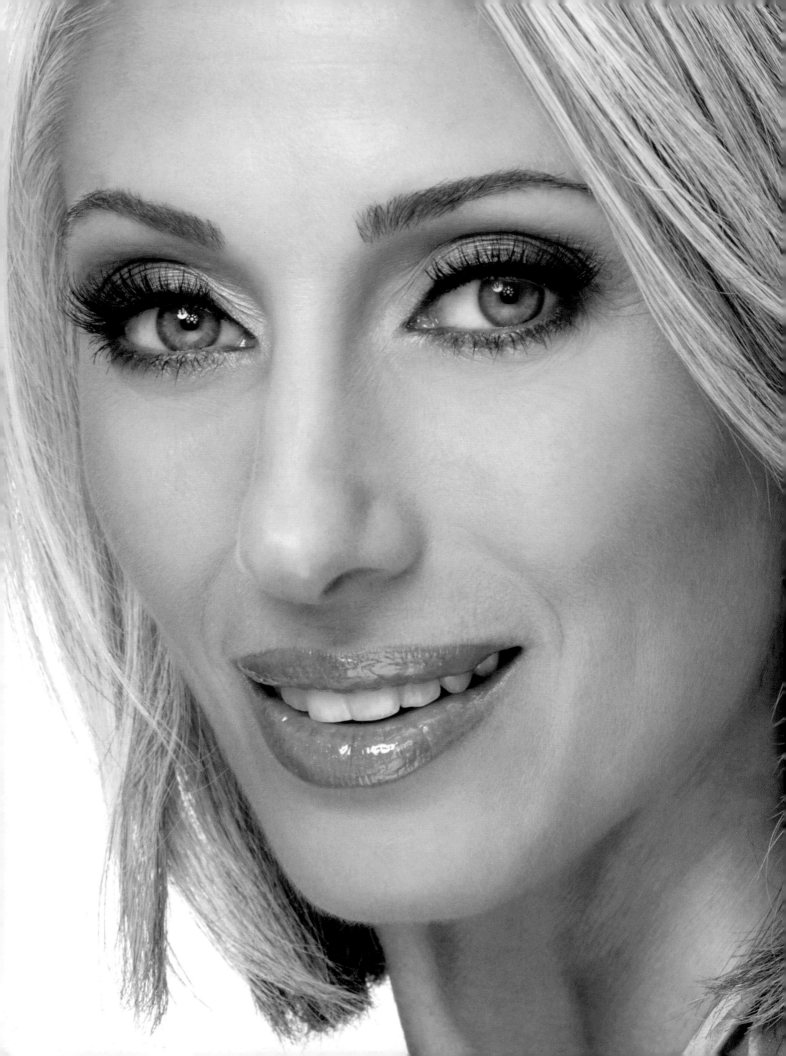

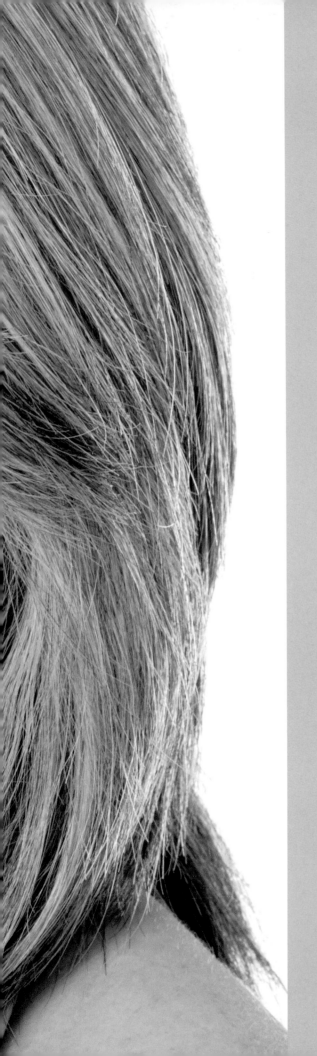

4

medically speaking

One major part of your face has a lot to do with how youthful you look: your skin. The appearance of your skin can hide or show your true age. We all know that a good skincare regimen is priceless, and I'll definitely get to that. But first, I want to discuss the major causes of skin aging and what you can do to prevent it.

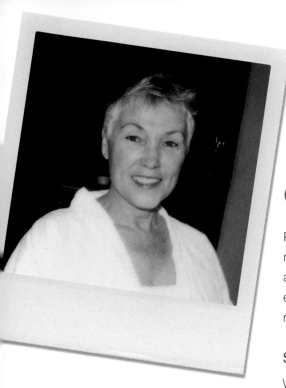

causes and prevention

Prevention is your first line of defense in doing battle against aging. In my research for this book, I found a wide variety of opinions, but after gathering all my research together and really studying it, I found three common aging enemies that almost all experts agree on: sun exposure, smoking, and the natural aging process.

sun exposure

We've all heard that sun is bad for your skin. Studies show that it causes photoaging and cancer. Photoaging is damage to the skin, such as wrinkles or discoloration, caused by prolonged exposure to sunlight.

The sun produces many different rays that damage your skin. The two main rays, or types of solar radiation, you need to know about are UVA and UVB rays (to keep the two rays straight, UV=ultraviolet, A=aging, and B= burning). UVB rays are the strongest and are the cause of sunburn; they can also lead to skin cancer. The SPF level (sun protection factor) of a product describes its effectiveness in blocking UVB rays.

UVA rays cause aging. They penetrate the deepest layers of the skin, causing darkening of skin pigment that can lead to spots, as well as dryness and wrinkles. Exposure to these light rays breaks down the skin's connective tissues, collagen and elastin. The destruction of these tissues results in a loss of strength and resilience in your skin, causing it to sag and wrinkle.

Your best line of defense is to do everything you can to prevent the damage from happening. You *must* wear sunscreen every day and stay out of the sun as much as possible. When in the sun for long periods of time, use a sunscreen with a higher SPF. I know you have heard this over and over, but it is true. General consensus within the medical industry suggests using a minimum of SPF 30 for everyday wear, but the higher, the better. Also, make sure that your sunscreen blocks both UVA and UVB rays. Cover any part of your skin that does not have to be exposed to the sun (repeat after me: long sleeves look nice, I love long sleeves).

smoking

As with sun exposure, smoking destroys collagen and elastin in the skin. Nicotine actually has a harmful effect on tiny blood vessels in your face that feed and nourish your skin. Most experts consider smoking the number one cause of premature aging. In addition to nicotine destroying collagen and causing a loss of elasticity, the recurring use of certain muscles around the mouth during smoking can cause deep creases. Some experts believe, as do I, that smoking can change the pigmentation of your skin, making it look dull and sallow. The best way to prevent these aging effects is to simply not smoke. Bottom line: Smoking is robbing you of beauty and youth.

aging

Yes, the ticking of the clock is not helping you look younger. Unfortunately, as you get older, your skin naturally thins and becomes less elastic. Genetics definitely plays a huge role in aging, and some people are luckier than others. But how you treat your skin through the years matters, too. Doing the right things can definitely slow the natural aging process. Not smoking, protecting your skin from the sun, and proper skincare can all contribute to a youthful look.

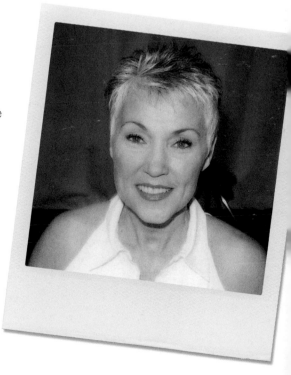

As you get older, your skin produces fewer natural oils, fat production in the deeper layers of the skin (which makes the skin look full and plump) lessens, and your skin loses its ability to retain as much moisture as it once did. To top it off, the rate at which your skin sheds old cells slows down. When you're thirty or younger, your skin regenerates about every twenty-five days, but after thirty, that regeneration slows. Dead cells build up on your skin and increase the appearance of fine lines. A buildup of these dead cells can make your skin look older—not what any woman wants!

Exfoliating, the process of removing or helping your skin to release these dead cells, is at the top of every expert's list of things that women can do to look younger. Exfoliating your skin is probably one of the fastest ways to give your skin a fresh look, and it also improves your skin tone. There are two types of exfoliation, mechanical and chemical.

A mechanical exfoliator contains grains or granules (natural or manmade) with a slightly abrasive texture that help remove dead cells mechanically. Chemical exfoliators are products that contain glycolic acid or alpha hydroxy acids (AHA), which loosen the cells that hold dead skin on the surface of your skin.

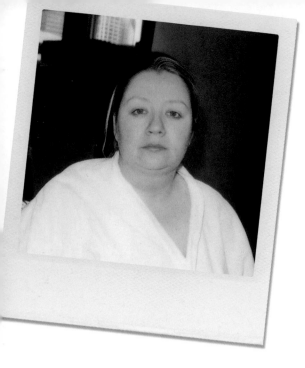

what to do

Proper skincare is your first defense in battling the signs of aging. It is important to start a good regimen as soon as possible! I can't recommend a definitive regime, because skincare is personal and everyone's needs are different. I will say, though, that your skin—and its needs—changes as you age. What works for you in your twenties probably won't work in your thirties. So, be prepared to make changes in your regime as your skin changes.

There are some key considerations when making good skincare choices, and they're based on your skin type. The type of cleanser, moisturizer, eye crème, toner, and mask you use is determined by whether your skin is dry, oily, or normal. Let's review the options.

cleanser

- **dry skin:** Choose a cleanser with a crème or oil base, which moisturizes as it cleanses and doesn't strip your skin of its natural oils.

- **oily skin:** Choose a water-based cleanser containing ingredients that absorb excess oil.

- **normal skin:** You can choose a cleanser with either base. Just be sure it doesn't strip your skin of its oils and isn't too high in detergent; it could irritate your skin.

moisturizer

- **dry skin:** To restore moisture to dry skin, choose a crème or oil-based moisturizer that contains urea or propylene glycol, chemicals that help keep your skin moist. For very dry, cracked skin, oils are preferable. They have more staying power than crèmes do and are more effective in preventing water from evaporating from your skin.

- **oily skin:** An oily complexion is prone to acne and breakouts. Although oily, such skin still needs moisture, especially after using skincare products that remove oils and dry out the skin. A light moisturizer can help protect your skin after washing. Be sure to pick an oil-free, water-based product and look for products labeled "noncomedogenic," which means they won't clog pores. Also look for moisturizers containing oil-absorbing ingredients, to further help your skin look fresh without appearing shiny.

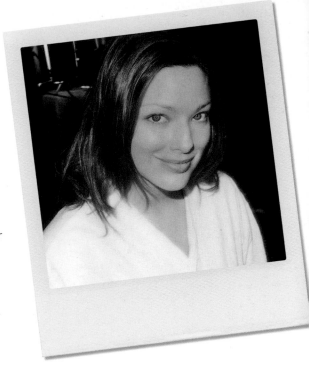

- **normal skin:** Lucky you, your skin is neither too dry nor too oily. To maintain this natural moisture balance, use a water-based moisturizer with a light, non-greasy feel. These moisturizers often contain light-weight oils, such as cetyl alcohol, or silicone-derived ingredients, such as cyclomethicone.

- **mature skin:** As you age, your skin tends to become drier because your oil-producing glands become less active. To keep your skin soft and well hydrated, choose an oil-based moisturizer with petrolatum as the base, along with lactic acid or alpha hydroxy acids. These ingredients help hold moisture and prevent flaky, scaly skin.

eye crème

The skin underneath the eyes is thinner and more delicate than other places on the face. Eye crèmes are specially formulated for this area. For daytime, use a lightweight eye crème that hydrates and absorbs into the skin; it helps keep the skin looking smoother and everything you apply over it looks and adheres better. For night, use a richer, more moisturizing formula.

toner

This product can give that little extra bit of cleansing: It will remove anything your cleanser might have left behind. Using toner helps keep pores completely clean. This step is not a must it is a choice, for those that want a little extra cleansing. It can also help close the pores after cleansing.

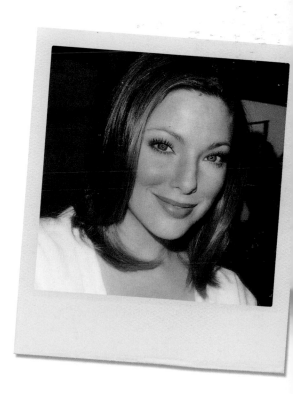

masks

- **clay masks:** A clay mask deep-cleans pores by drawing out impurities and any extra dirt (which helps prevent blackheads). It's great for oily skin.

- **hydrating masks:** These masks add extra moisture to the skin, giving an extra boost to really dry, aging skin.an extra boost to really dry, aging skin.

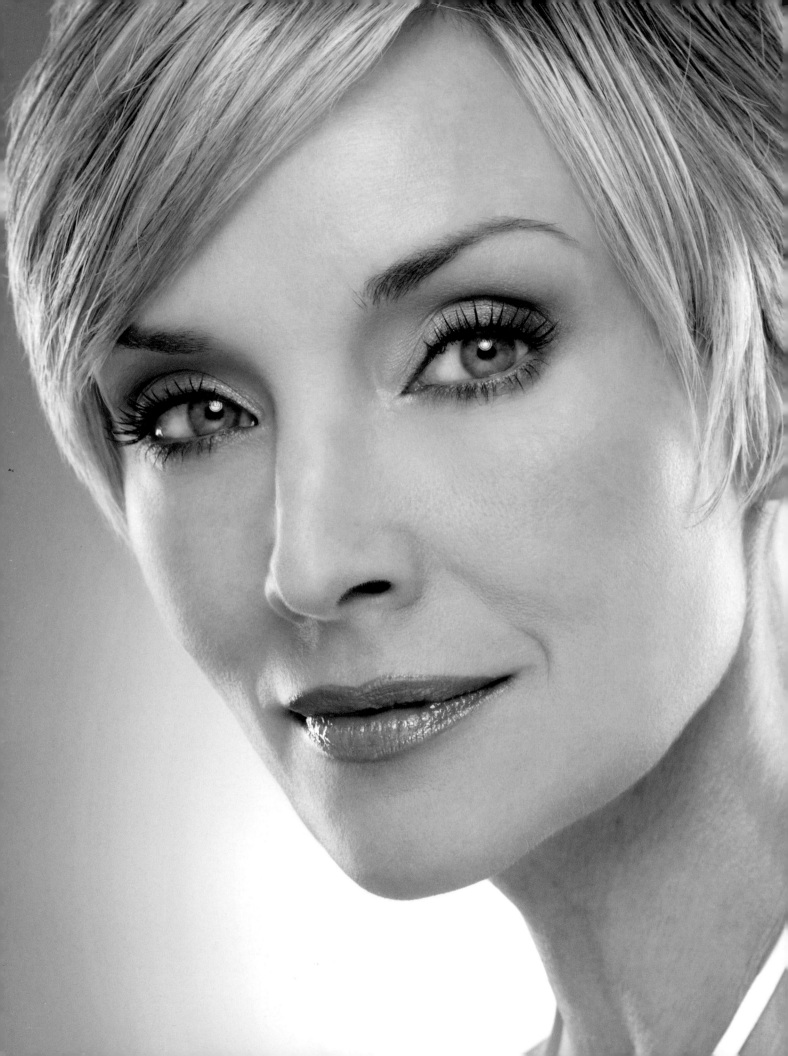

possible options

If wrinkles and deep creases bother you, you have many options to minimize their appearance. Treatments vary in invasiveness and intensity. There are medications that will give you more subtle results than medical procedures, and other techniques that can give you more dramatic results. Here's a quick overview:

medications

Topical medications that you apply to your skin are less expensive (but less dramatic) than surgical procedures. The most effective are retinoids, the so-called "wrinkle creams," and hydroquinones.

- **retinoids:** Derived from vitamin A, retinoids, when applied to your skin, can reduce the appearance of fine wrinkles, splotchy pigmentation, and skin roughness. Retinoids must be used with a skincare program that includes sunscreen and protective clothing, because the medication can make your skin burn easily. It may also cause redness, dryness, itching, and a burning or tingling sensation. Tretinoin (Renova, Retin-A) and tazarotene (Avage, Tazorac) are examples of topical retinoids.

- **nonprescription wrinkle creams:** The effectiveness of anti-wrinkle creams depends in part on the active ingredient or ingredients. Retinol, alpha hydroxy acids, kinetin, copper peptides, coenzyme Q10, and antioxidants may result in improvements in the appearance of wrinkles. However, nonprescription wrinkle creams contain lower concentrations of active ingredients than prescription creams do.

- **hydroquinones:** This product is prescribed to help bleach the skin, reducing the appearance of dark spots, age spots, and hyperpigmentation.

medical procedures and other techniques

A variety of resurfacing techniques, injectables, fillers, and surgical procedures is available to smooth out wrinkles and fine lines. Each works differently and has its own degree of effectiveness and results.

- **dermabrasion:** This procedure involves sanding down (planing) the surface layer of your skin with a rapidly rotating brush. The planing removes the skin surface and a new layer of skin grows in its place.

- **microdermabrasion:** This technique is similar to dermabrasion, but less surface skin is removed. It's done using a vacuum suction over your face while aluminum oxide crystals essentially sandblast your skin. Only a fine layer of skin is removed.

- **photo facial:** An IPL (Intense Pulsed Light) Photo Facial is a series of full-face, pulsed-light treatments intended to reduce the appearance of fine lines, sun damage, and aged skin. An intense light is emitted in a series of gentle pulses over the entire face.

- **laser resurfacing:** In this technique, a laser beam is used to destroy the outer layer of skin (epidermis) and heat the underlying skin (dermis), which stimulates the growth of new collagen. As the skin heals, new skin forms that is smoother and tighter. It can take up to several months to fully heal from laser resurfacing. Less-intense lasers (nonablative lasers), pulsed light sources, and radio frequency devices don't injure the epidermis. These treatments heat the dermis and cause new collagen and elastin formation. After several treatments, the skin feels firmer and appears refreshed.

- **alpha-hydroxy peel:** This is a mixture of alpha-hydroxy acids, such as glycolic, lactic, and fruit acids, which are applied to the skin to even out skin texture and reduce superficial wrinkles. Ten-percent-strength peels can be performed by aestheticians in a spa.

- **chemical peel:** With this technique, an acid is applied to the target areas, which burns the outer layer of your skin. With medium-depth peels, the entire epidermis and a small portion of the dermis are removed. New skin forms to take its place. The new skin is usually smoother and less wrinkled than the old skin. Redness lasts up to several months. With superficial peels, only a portion of the epidermis is removed. After a series of peels, you may notice fewer fine lines and fading of brown spots.

- **botox:** When injected in small doses into specific muscles, Botox prevents the muscles from contracting or flexing. When the muscles cannot tighten or flex, the skin stays flat and appears smooth and less wrinkled. Botox works well on frown lines between the eyebrows, across the forehead, and on wrinkles in the outer corners of the eyes.

- **soft tissue fillers:** Soft tissue fillers, which include fat, collagen, and hyaluronic acid (Restylane, Juvederm), can be injected into deeper wrinkles on your face. They plump and smooth out wrinkles and furrows and give the skin more volume.

- **collagen injections:** Small amounts of collagen are injected directly into areas where they're needed. They raise the skin in depressed or recessed areas of the face, minimizing facial lines and scars. A skin test is required one month in advance to determine if a patient is eligible for treatment with collagen, because some patients can experience an allergic reaction to the injections.

I am not suggesting that you need one or more of these services or medications! But I wanted to introduce the available options. Any of them can freshen up your skin and possibly give your skin a more youthful appearance.

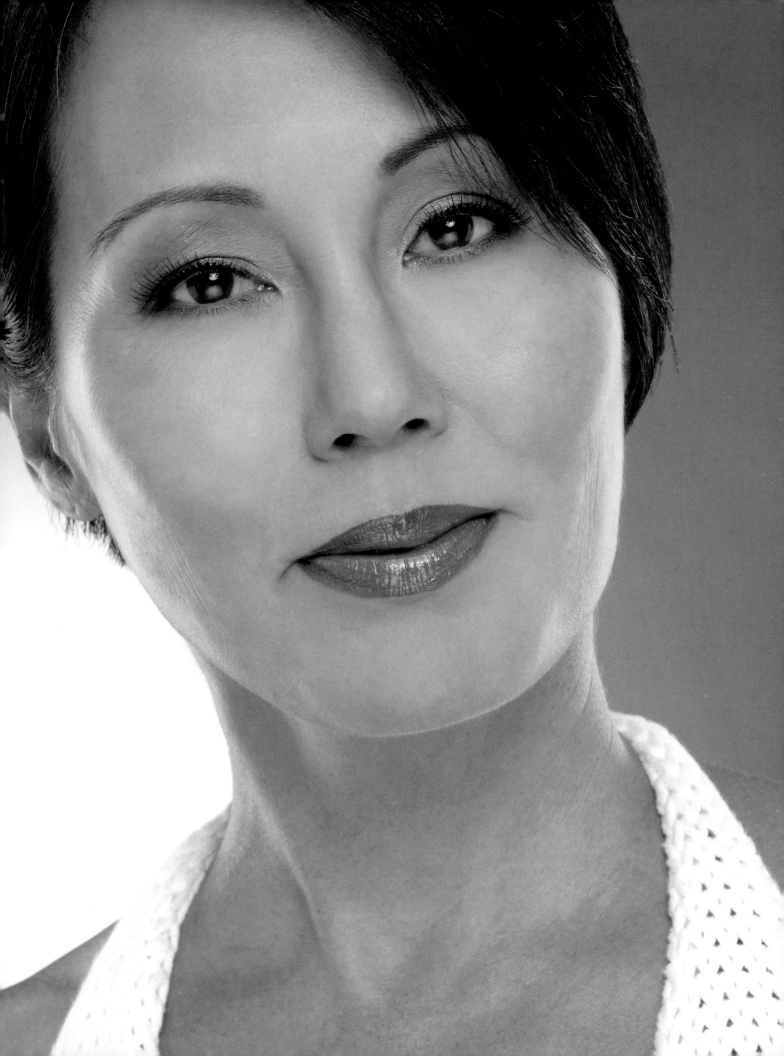

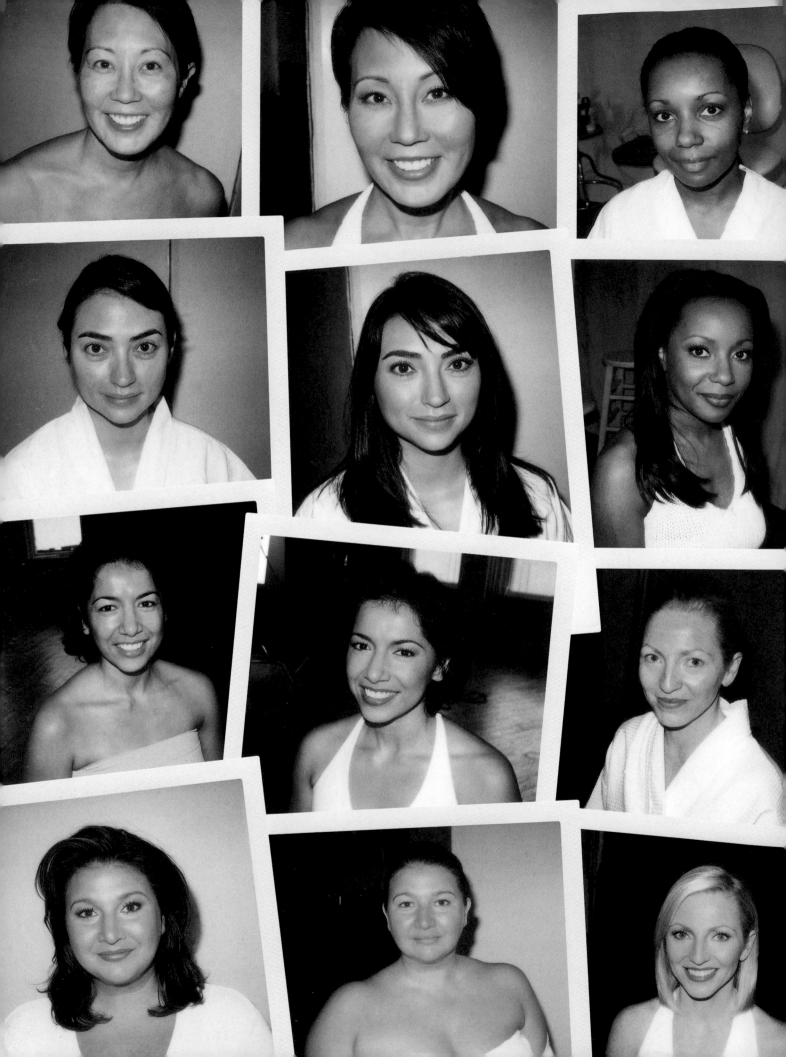

part two | bringing out your youthful beauty

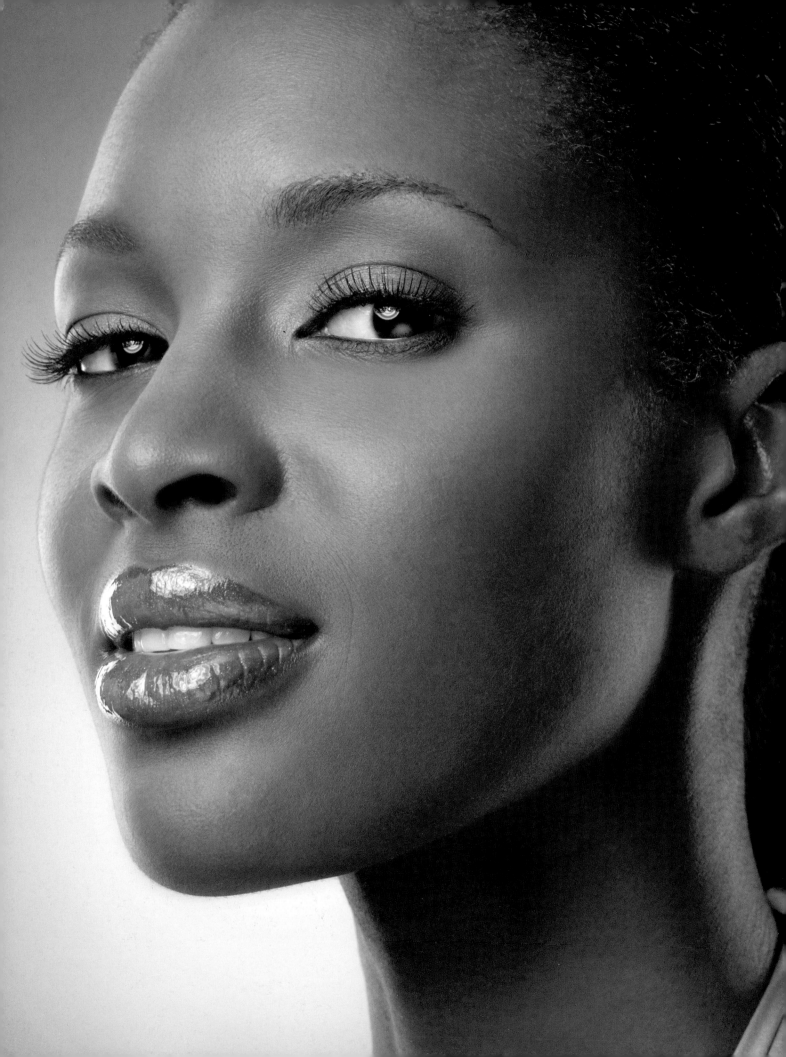

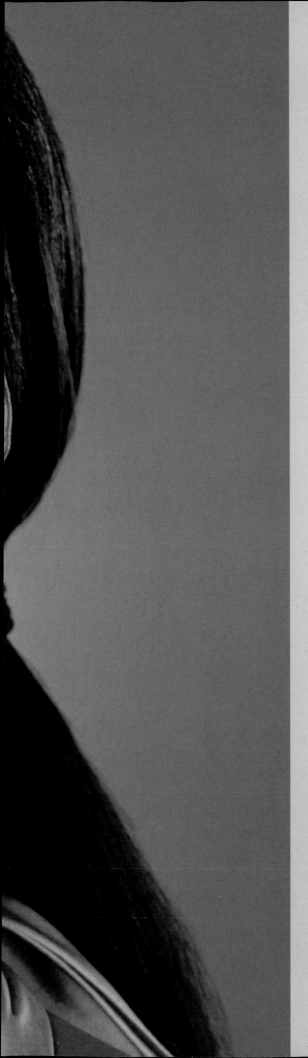

5

preparing
for perfection

A big part of looking younger is taking the right
steps and making the right choices to achieve
your goal. Before you start to apply the great
makeup choices you have already made, believe
it or not, you need to do a little prep work. You
can choose the perfect foundation, concealer,
eyeshadow, blush, and lipstick, but if your skin
and face aren't ready for them, they will do you no
good. With that in mind, achieving a flawless finish
and application begins with a few simple tricks
up front. From exquisitely arched eyebrows to skin
that has been perfectly prepped for makeup, great
results do not require a lot of effort, just a little
prep work.

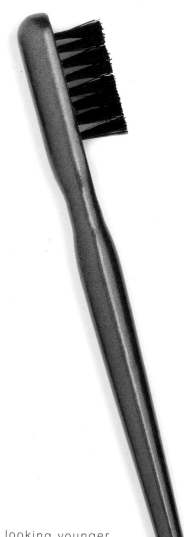

youthful brows

Well-groomed eyebrows are a must for anyone, but they're even more important if you want to look younger. They can make such a difference! Brows are the picture frames of your eyes. The right brow shape can actually lift your face and open up your eyes.

Before you reach for the tweezers, however, please take some professional advice: You should embrace your natural brow shape, because no matter how much you tweeze, you cannot turn your brows into something they are not. Some brows naturally curve into a gentle arch; others grow straight across. However your brows grow, you need to shape them to suit the way they grow on your face. But have no fear! Whatever their shape, we can groom them to flatter your features.

Let me start by sharing two more key points with you. First, fuller brows make you look younger—honestly, they do. So do not over-tweeze your brows; you want them to look naturally full. If you have already over-tweezed, no worries—visit page 158 to learn how to make them look thicker. Second, do not follow fashion trends. The trend will change, and you will be left with brows that are not right for your face. Always shape your brows to suit your face and the way they naturally grow.

Before we begin, gather your tools. You will need a good pair of tweezers, a brow brush, and a small pair of scissors. Now, we're ready to start! Let's begin by evaluating your brows. Are they too dense? Trimming can soften eyebrows that are too dense or heavy. It can completely change the way the brow hairs lie on the face.

trimming

Often, brow hairs are actually longer than they appear, because the tips of the hairs are lighter in color, and when they reach a certain length, they tend to curl. Trimming them removes some of the density and that slight curl, so that the hairs lie more neatly.

To trim your brow hairs, simply brush them up and snip any stray hairs that extend past the upper brow line. Next, brush them down and snip any unruly hairs that extend past the lower brow line. Now brush them back into place. Notice how much better they lie and how much softer they look on your face.

If you need to trim your brows, it should be done before you start to tweeze. You don't want to ruin your brow line by tweezing away hairs that should have stayed but were simply too long.

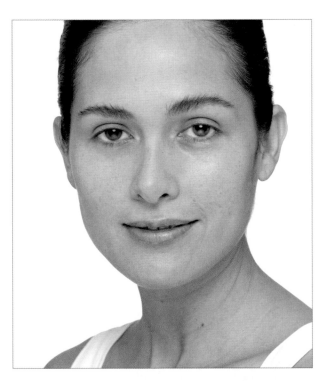

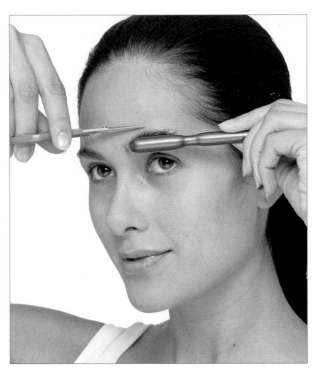

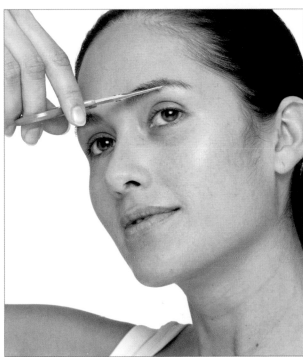

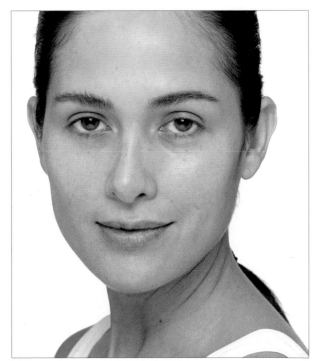

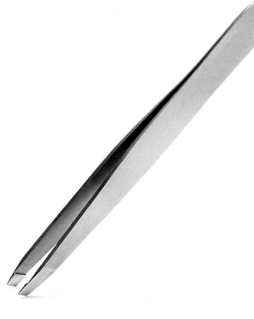

tweezing

Now it's time to tweeze.

The best time to tweeze your brows is after a steamy shower. It's a lot less painful then, because your pores are already open. Try to tweeze in natural light. You can better see what you're doing. Always tweeze in the same direction as the hair grows. Tweezing in the opposite direction can damage the hair follicle, and the hair might not grow back properly—sticking straight out, for example, rather than lying down.

If you are born with naturally full brows, you never want to tweeze them pencil-thin; your face needs a fuller brow. Shape them and groom them, just do not over-tweeze them.

Tweezing your brows to match each other can be very difficult. Very few women have brows that grow identically. You can tweeze one brow and never make the other brow match the first one, no matter how you tweezed. If, instead, you do what I call "tweezing side to side," you can tweeze your brows more evenly. Start by tweezing a couple of hairs out of one brow, then switch to the other brow and tweeze a couple out of it, then switch back to the first. By switching brows with every tweeze, you can constantly reevaluate what needs to be tweezed, and the frequent comparison will help you get them more even.

tips:

When tweezing, be sure to tweeze one hair at a time. Tweezing clusters can cause bald spots.

Take care not to overdo it, because sparse brows, especially on a mature face, make the face look older. Fuller brows make you look younger.

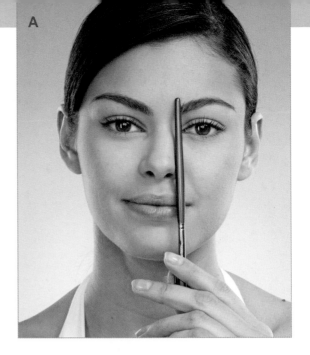

how do you determine where to start?

You will know where and what to tweeze by using three key points of reference. Simply follow these directions for perfect brows.

point A. Hold a pencil or the handle of a brush vertically against the side of your nose and notice where it meets the brow. This is where your brow should begin.

point B. Hold the pencil against your nostril and move it diagonally across the outer half of the iris of your eye. Notice where the pencil meets the brow. This is the best place for the peak of your arch. If you tweeze from Point A to Point B, tapering the line slightly toward the peak, you will create the ideal shape for your brow. It is a gentle taper, starting with the natural width at the beginning of your brow (point A) and slowly tapering thinner as you get to the arch (point B).

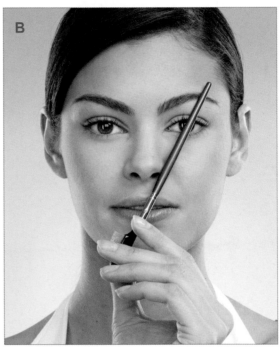

point C. Again, place the pencil against your nostril, but this time, extend it diagonally to the outer corner of your eye. Where it meets the brow is the best place for your brow to end. If you tweeze from Point B to Point C, tapering the line even thinner, you will create the best brow shape for your face. Once again, it is a slow taper from point B to point C, not a drastic change.

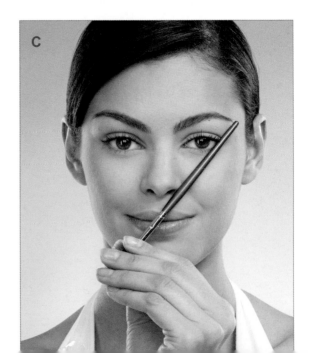

"fuller brows make you look younger"

I have been trying to grow my brows back in to look fuller, but it seems that no matter what I do, they are not getting any thicker. What can—or should—I do?

To help your brows grow back in, you must leave them alone and tweeze nothing for at least a couple of months. By tweezing, you can tweeze out what you think is an unnecessary hair, which, in reality, might be needed when your brows fill in. You must leave them alone completely, so that they can fill in. You can also turn to some new products that help promote new hair growth. Thanks to new technology, you can grow back hairs that you thought were gone for good. Check our website www.robertjonesbeauty.com for products.

I have heard so many different opinions about waxing my eyebrows. Should I, or shouldn't I?

You can wax unwanted hairs, but be aware that the hairs may not grow back correctly, because the wax is pulled off in the opposite direction of the hairs' growth, and that can damage the hair follicle. Also, I feel that waxing repeatedly may eventually give a crepe-like appearance to the skin. Now that is just my opinion, but every time you rip off hot wax, you also take off a layer of skin. And, if you have ever been waxed with wax that is too hot, you *know* it will take off skin. So, if you want to have your brows waxed, I say, find a salon that uses a non-heated wax. There are cold waxes that can get the job done. A great alternative is to have your brows threaded, a process in which your brows are shaped using a thread. Call your local salons and ask if they thread.

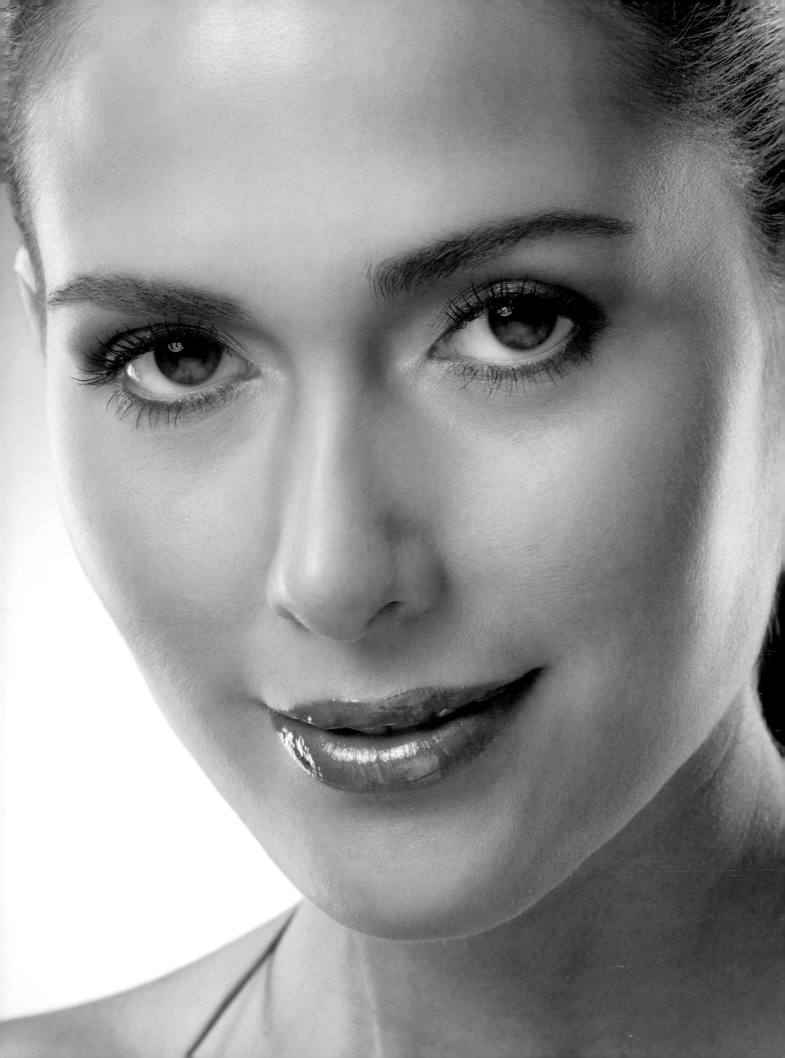

sunni, 30s

Sunni is so beautiful, but I had to do something about those dark circles. What a difference. I love that I was able to narrow her nose and give her such a beautiful glow.

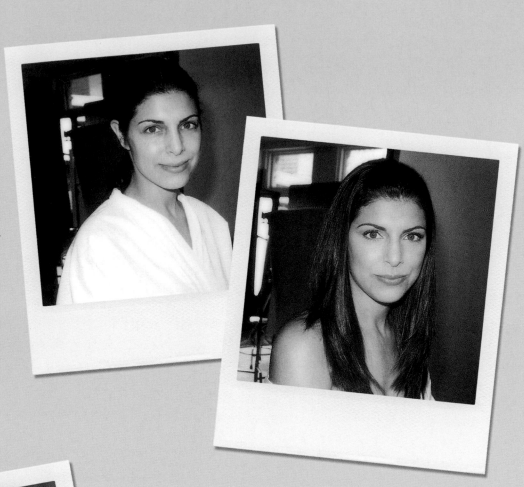

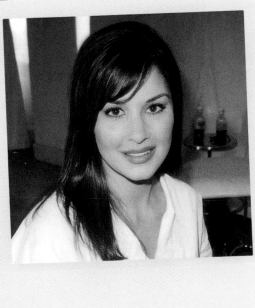

natalie, 30s

I love Natalie's square face, and she has beautiful eyes. I'm pleased that I was able to really draw attention to her eyes.

moisturizer

Moisturizing is especially important to achieve younger-looking skin. It's the first step in preparing your skin for everything else you are about to apply. Without it, you will never get the flawless application that you want and deserve. Moisturizer evens out the porosity of your skin, so that everything that follows adheres evenly and smoothly. Regardless of your skin type, even if it's oily, you need to start with moisturizer. Just remember to choose the correct type for your skin's needs. See page 66 to review which formula is best for your skin.

Be sure to begin with a freshly washed face, then apply your moisturizer. It's best applied to a damp face, because it goes on more evenly. Warm a quarter-sized amount of moisturizer with your fingertips, then blend it over your entire face and neck (don't forget the neck!). Moisturizer is most effective when it's left to absorb for a few minutes before you apply your makeup. It must be completely dry before you apply anything else—if it isn't, products applied afterward won't adhere evenly.

While you're waiting for the moisturizer to be absorbed, apply your eye crème and lip balm, so they to have time to absorb before you apply anything over them.

tip:

As you get older, your lids can become dry and crepey. But you should never apply moisturizer or eye crème to the eyelids before you put on eyeshadow, because it will cause the shadow to crease and not last as long. If you want to moisturize your lids, do it before bed, not in the morning.

primer

Primer is one of my *looking younger* secret weapons. It's an optional makeup step that can do wonders for your skin's appearance. This is a product that you might not know a lot about. Primer seals in your moisturizer and helps your foundation go on more evenly and last longer. It can improve the look of your skin and keep it looking fresh all day. Primer prevents foundation and concealer from seeping into fine lines and keeps your skin's natural oils from altering your foundation color, by creating a barrier between them. It sometimes contains light-reflecting properties that help diminish the appearance of small flaws. Apply it just like you would a moisturizer, after your moisturizer and before your foundation.

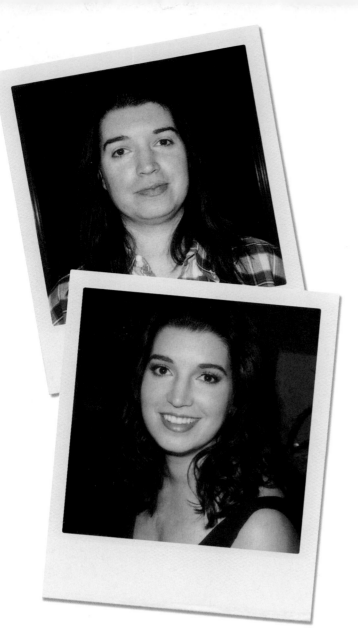

exfoliate

Exfoliating your lips regularly can keep them looking fresh and luscious and your lip texture smooth and soft. A perfect time to do this is right after you shower. Apply a generous amount of lip balm and wait a few minutes for it to absorb. Using a soft-bristle toothbrush, brush your lips vigorously, then apply more lip balm. If you prefer, you can use a towel to rub your lips instead of a brush. Regardless of the method you use, always moisturize when you're finished. Exfoliating your lips regularly also helps your lipstick go on more smoothly and your lips appear younger and smoother.

kristy, 30s

I wanted to lift Kristy's eyes and open them up, to make them her focus. This is proof of what a difference the right eye makeup can make. What a beauty.

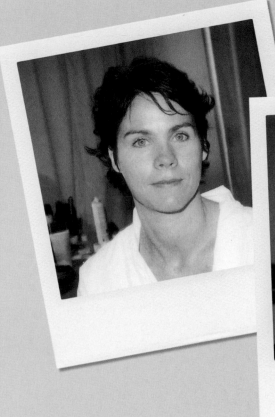

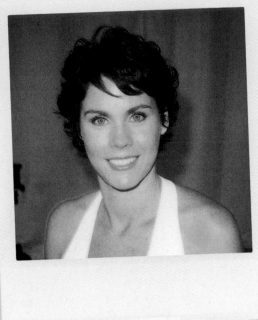

jamie, 40s

Look at those beautiful blue eyes. The right shades of eyeshadow really brought out the blue.

susan, 30s

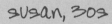

All I could see was Susan's beautiful smile. I was pleased that I could really draw attention to it. Looking at her after I was finished makes me want to smile.

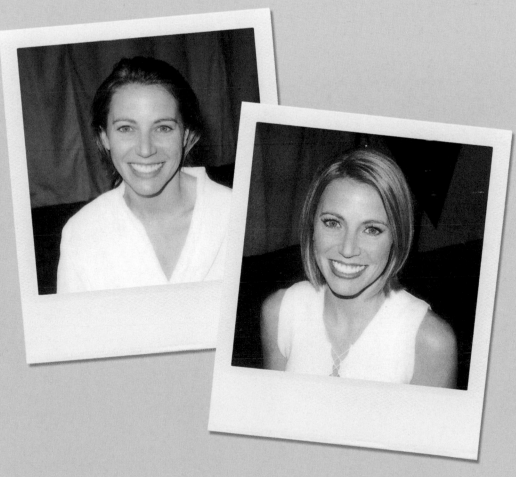

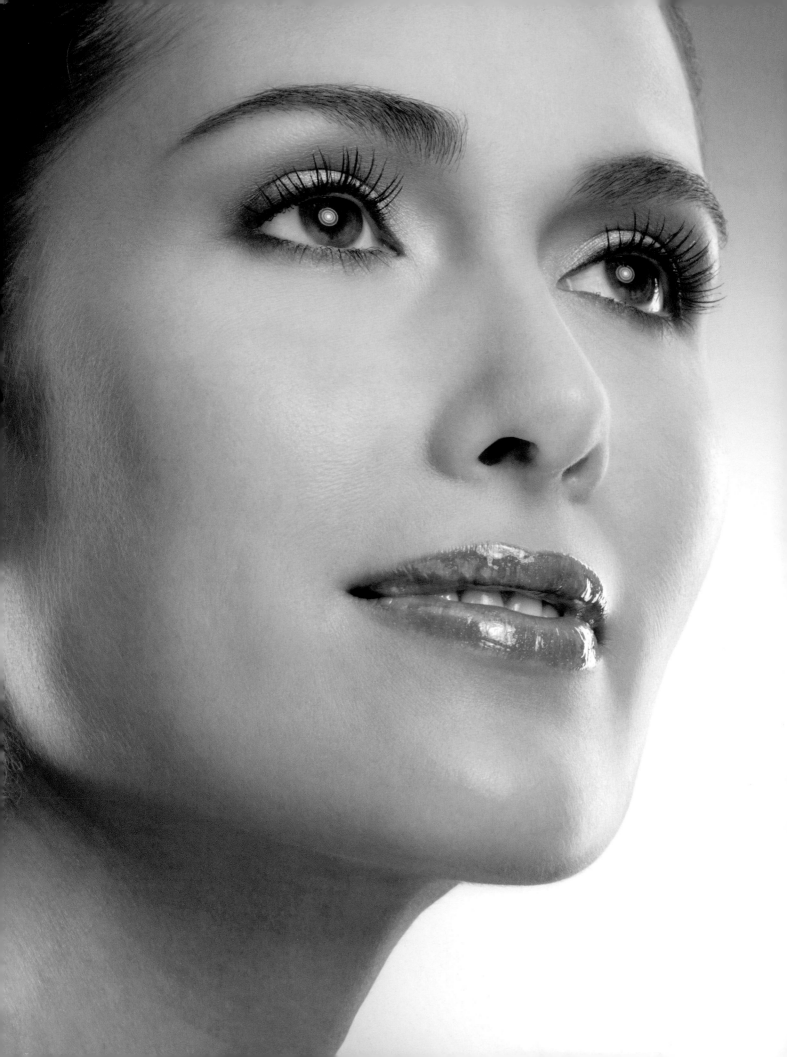

6

creating flawless skin

Looking younger is our goal, and one of the best ways to achieve that goal is to create flawless-looking skin. Studies have shown that most people associate age with discoloration and uneven skin tone. In one study, women with spots or skin flaws were perceived as being much older than those with flawless skin. So, in this chapter, we'll learn how to create the illusion of flawless, younger-looking skin.

Before I show you how to cover your flaws, let me remind you that practice makes perfect. Don't expect to always get it right the first time you try a new technique! You might need to try things two or three times. If you try a technique and it doesn't work, just wash it off and try again.

Now, I want to be realistic: "flawless" is subjective. I can't make you look twelve, but I can certainly help you look your youngest. You can learn to cover the things you do not want to see. Read through this chapter; when we're finished, you will be an expert at making yourself look younger *and* more beautiful. Play and practice—that's how to perfect your application techniques. Now, let's start looking younger!

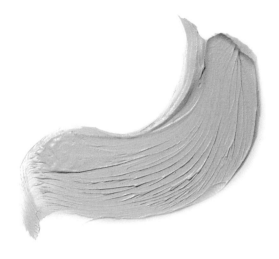

foundation

The first step in achieving flawless-looking skin is choosing the right foundation. Many women find this hard to do, so don't feel like a failure if you're one of them. Wearing the wrong shade of foundation can actually make you look older, so I definitely want to help you choose the right shade—our goal, after all, is to help you look younger! In this section, I will give you all the information you need to help you pick the perfect shade and formula of foundation.

choosing foundation

Following is a short list of questions to ask yourself when choosing foundation. Your answers will help you find the perfect match.

1. What color is the undertone of my skin—olive, yellow, pink, golden orange, or warm brown?
2. What is the depth level of my skin—from very pale porcelain all the way to very deep ebony?
3. What is my skin type—oily, dry, combination, or normal?
4. How much coverage do I want from my foundation—sheer, medium, or full?
5. What type of finish do I want my foundation to give my skin—matte, satin, dewy, or luminous?

Before we get started answering these questions, however, I first want to make things easier by placing all women into two basic skin tone categories: ivory/beige and bronze/ebony. The reason for doing this is because, even though most of what we will be discussing is the same for both, there are a few things we need to think about that are specific to each separate skin tone category.

I want to make it clear that the only way to get an exact shade match for your foundation is to do a stripe test. Let me repeat: Stripe-testing is the *only* way to get an exact match. Convinced? Good. Let's try it now. Here are a few rules to follow:

1. Always conduct your stripe test in natural light.
2. Try several shades, until you find the perfect match.
3. The shade that matches your neck is the right shade.

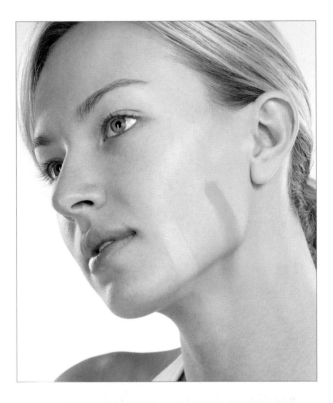

ivory/beige

If you have ivory/beige skin tones, conduct the stripe test from your jaw down onto your neck, because you want to match your neck. Women with ivory/beige skin tend to have redness in their faces, but not in their necks, so it's important to get a true match for the neck. Although you do not want to apply foundation to your neck—only to your face—it is imperative that it match your neck, so you can stop your application at your jawline. Start by applying stripes of three different foundation shades from your jaw to your neck, then wait a few minutes to see if the oils in your skin change the pigments. Select the one that most closely matches your neck.

bronze/ebony

Women with bronze/ebony skin tones should stripe-test from their cheek down to their jaw, because some women with these skin tones (some, not most, not even close to most, but some) have what is called facial masking (skin that is darker at the outer edges of the face and lighter in the interior area of the face) and we must go across both shades of skin to get the perfect match. Start by applying stripes of three different foundation shades extending from your cheek to your jaw area, and wait a few minutes to see if the oils in your skin change the pigments. Select the one that most closely matches your neck.

If you have any degree of facial masking, I suggest using my technique of applying two shades of foundation to perfect your skin tone: one shade to brighten your skin, and another to deepen it. Turn to page 102 to find out why two shades are better than one when it comes to facial masking and how to apply them.

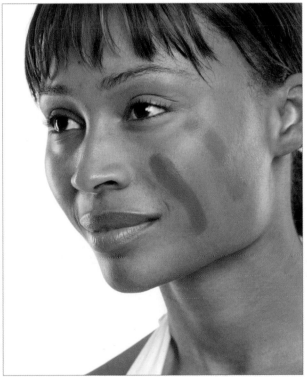

Q&A

Whenever I try to get a perfect match for my foundation, the lighting in the store makes it impossible to tell if the shade is correct or not. How can I make sure it matches?

When stripe-testing in a department store, carry a mirror with you, so you can walk outside into natural daylight to see which shade is your perfect match. If you buy foundation at your local drugstore, where you obviously can't try the shades on your skin, bring a mirror with you, then take three shades you think most closely match your skin and walk to the nearest window. Hold each bottle close to your face to see which one is the closest match. If you are not sure, you could always buy the two that look the closest and mix them to get your perfect shade.

It seems like I can never find the perfect shade! When I compare shades, one always seems a little too light and one a little too dark. Which should I choose?

If you are choosing between two shades and one seems a little too light, while the other one seems a little too dark, choose the slightly darker shade. The lighter shade will only make you look older. Just apply it with a light hand and blend really well along your jawline.

what is the undertone of your skin?

This is probably the single most difficult thing for a woman to determine. When looking at your face and neck, it is sometimes hard to see your true undertone, because of possible discoloration from sun and other irritants. But there is another place you can look to see your true undertone: the inside of your arm. You do not stripe-test there because it is usually paler than your face and neck, but you can look there to see your skin's true undertone. The inside of your arm is less prone to discoloration, so it's easier to determine your skin's undertone from there than trying to guess from your face or neck. Why is the undertone so important? The first step to looking younger is choosing the right undertone for your foundation.

Let's go through both skin tone categories and learn how to figure out your undertone.

"the first step to looking younger is choosing the right undertone for your foundation"

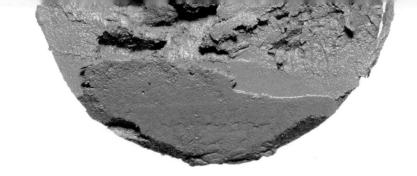

ivory/beige

If you have ivory/beige skin, you will have one of three basic undertones: olive, yellow, or pink. One of the most common mistakes women with ivory/beige skin make is choosing a foundation with a pink undertone. This will actually age you, because the pink undertone makes your skin look ashy and old. Many women think the pink undertone adds color to their skin, when, in fact, it does the opposite. The only women who need a pink undertone are women with pink in their face and neck.

Most women with ivory/beige skin benefit from a foundation with a yellow or olive undertone, because many with pink in their faces do not have any pink in their necks, and the goal is always to match the neck. Also, a foundation with a yellow or olive undertone adds color and life to the skin, making you look younger.

If you can't see your undertone, you can ask yourself the following question; it can help you determine your undertone. It is not an end-all, but it might help lead you in the right direction. Ask yourself: Do I tan easily? If the answer is yes, then you probably need a shade with an olive undertone, because what it takes to tan is olive pigment in your skin. If the answer is, "I don't know about easily (I might even burn a little first), but I can get a tan," then your skin probably has a yellow undertone. If your answer is, "I always burn rather than tan when I go out in the sun," then your skin probably has a pink undertone.

Yellow foundations can counteract the redness caused by skin conditions, such as rosacea and broken capillaries. Women with these conditions or with ruddy skin tones often feel that foundations with a yellow undertone look too yellow, because they're used to seeing red in their faces. Give it time! Your skin will start to absorb the foundation and work with it better, and your eye will get used to seeing the red neutralized. You'll soon notice a more even, natural, younger-looking skin.

bronze/ebony

Women with bronze/ebony skin should match the undertones in their skin exactly, because their undertones are so distinct and noticeable. They can range from yellow to golden orange to true brown. It is also quite possible for many bronze/ebony women to have multiple shades of skin on their face: lighter areas above the eyebrows and in the cheek area, for example, with darker areas around the mouth and along the jaw. You should never be afraid to use multiple shades of foundation—it can really even out your skin. Be sure to apply the correct shade of foundation only to the appropriate shade of skin (if you don't, it won't even out your skin). If there is a drastic difference between the center of your face and the outer area of your face, you might have facial masking. If so, visit page 102 to see how to even out your skin.

If you have very deep bronze/ebony skin, you might benefit from brightening (not lightening) your skin. When I say brightening, I mean this: After you have applied your appropriate foundation shade, apply a shade of foundation that is one or two shades lighter (in depth) than your natural shade and blend it into the center of your face (center of your forehead, underneath your eyes on top of your cheek bones, and tip of the chin). This will give you just a slight but very youthful glow, really waking up the appearance of your skin. Foundations with an intense golden orange undertone really work well for brightening bronze/ebony skin. You can achieve a more subtle version of this effect by using a powder to do the same thing. (Bear in mind that this technique works best on women whose skin is a darker shade of bronze/ebony.)

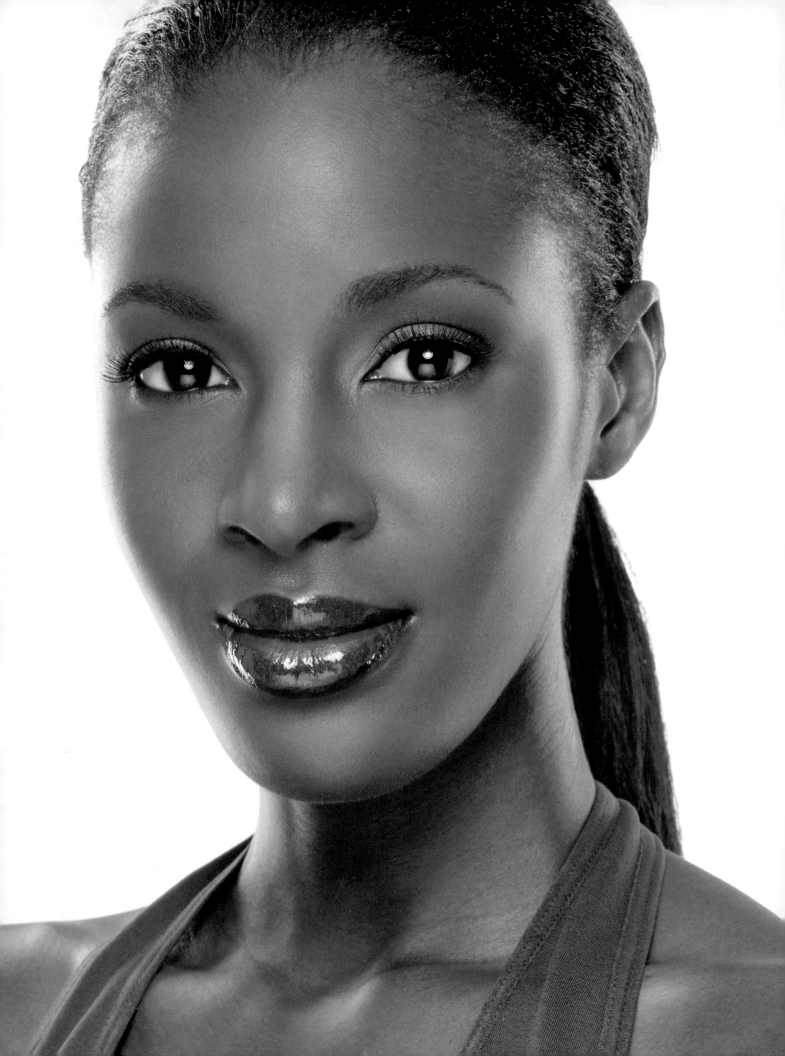

what is the depth level of your skin?

The depth level of your skin is how light or dark it appears to the naked eye. The paler your skin, the lighter its depth level; the darker your skin, the deeper its depth level. It is not only important to match your skin's undertone, you also want to match your skin's depth level. Choosing a foundation that is too light can actually make you look older. But you also don't want to choose a shade that is darker than your natural depth level, because it will make your skin look muddy and dirty.

what is your skin type?

It is important to know this, because you need to use the appropriate formula of foundation to go with your skin type. The right formula can make a huge difference in making you look younger and in helping your foundation stay in place all day. If your skin type is dry and you use a foundation containing no moisturizers, it can accentuate your fine lines (because of the lack of moisture). Your dry skin can also absorb the foundation, because it's trying to get all the moisture it needs. The result is foundation that disappears during the day, instead of one that lasts.

If your skin type is oily, using a formula without oil absorbers in it (to absorb the excess oil your skin secretes) can age your appearance by drawing attention to facial texture flaws, such as large pores and uneven skin texture. Remember, flawless skin makes you look younger!

If you have combination skin, I suggest using a foundation with oil absorbers to keep your t-zone (center of forehead, nose, cheeks, and chin) from getting too shiny and accentuating textural flaws. Women with normal skin should choose a foundation formula with a bit of moisture in it, to keep the skin moist and supple, healthy and youthful.

tips:

The best way to keep shine away on oily skin and avoid accentuating fine lines is to use blotting papers to absorb excess oil before you powder. When you use blotting papers, you need less powder to eliminate shine.

If you have an extreme combination skin type—very oily *and* very dry—don't be afraid to use two formulas of foundation, one with oil absorbers for the oily areas and one with moisturizers for the dry areas. This way, you give your skin exactly what it needs, where it needs it.

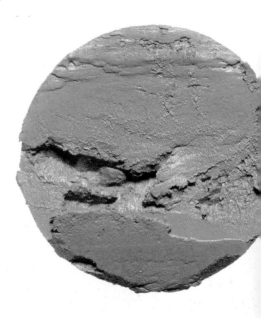

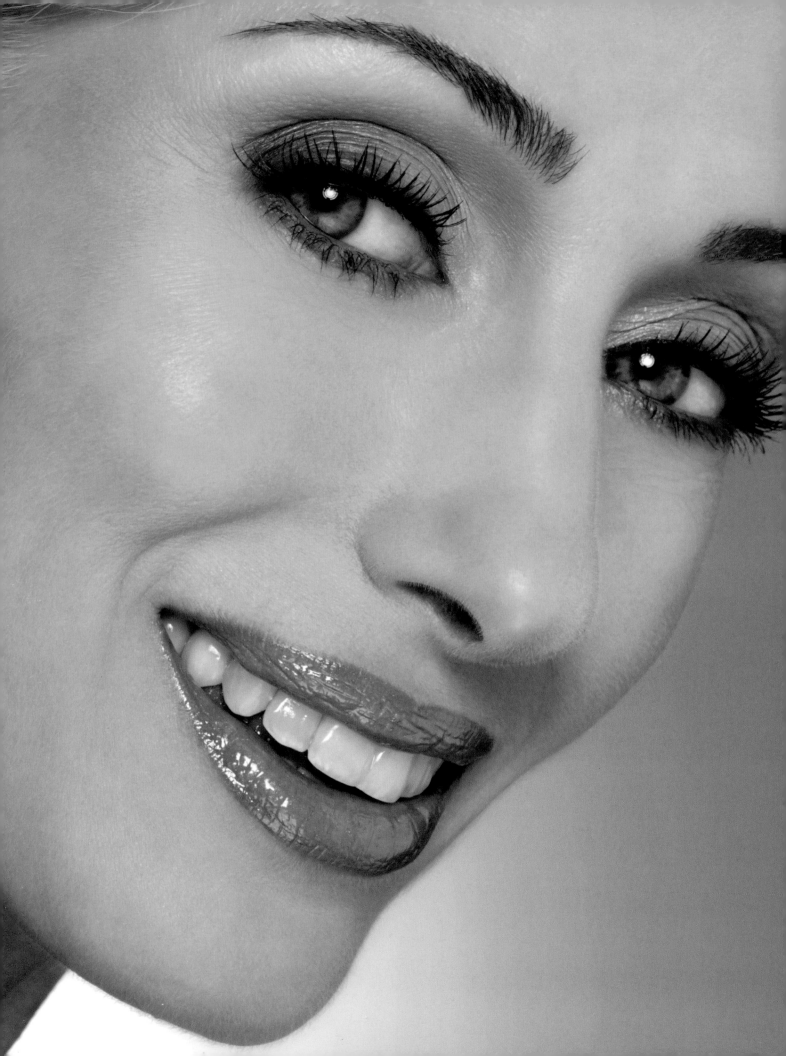

skin type chart

This skin-type chart helps explain at a glance the different skin types, their characteristics, what they need, and which foundation formulas are best for each.

skin type	characteristics	needs	best foundation
dry	lacks emollients; less elastic; rarely breaks out; feels tight after cleansing; usually small pores; mature skin (very often)	moisturizing foundations; formulas containing emollients and antioxidants	liquid (moisturizing); mousse; tinted moisturizer
normal	neither too oily nor too dry; smooth and even texture; medium to small pores; few to no breakouts; healthy color	pH-balanced products	liquid (all types); crème (all types); mousse; tinted moisturizer; dual-finish; mineral powder
oily	gets shiny fast; usually highly elastic; large pores; can break out often; prone to blackheads; wrinkles less	oil-free products; noncomedogenics; products enriched with oil absorbers	liquid (oil-free); mousse; crème-to-powder; dual-finish; mineral powder
sensitive	sensitive to many products; burns easily; flushes easily; blotchy (can have dry patches); susceptible to rosacea; thin and delicate	hypoallergenic; fragrance-free moisturizing formulas; formulas without chemical sunscreens	liquid (water-based); mousse; tinted moisturizer; dual-finish; mineral powder

"the smoother the skin, the more youthful it will appear"

how much coverage do you want?

The amount of coverage you need is determined by a combination of personal preference (do you feel more comfortable with more or less coverage?) and what you need to look flawless. Remember, the sheerer the foundation, the more natural it will look. But you need enough coverage to cover flaws you do not want to see. Consult Chapter 3 (page 29) for help in determining which foundation will work with your skin type and give you the coverage you want.

I need a little more coverage for some areas of my face, but I do not want to wear a foundation with heavier coverage over my entire face. What are my options?

To get the coverage you need, without using a heavy foundation all over your face, you can use two formulas. Apply a sheer formula first, then use a formula that provides heavier coverage in your problem areas. This can also reduce the amount of concealer you need, too. And the less concealer needed, the younger your skin will look.

My foundation does not seem to work year-round. Is this just my imagination?

This is definitely not just your imagination. Your skin can change from season to season (summer to winter). It also changes from year to year, as our skin ages. Your skin's depth level can be different in summer than in winter, so you might need a slightly deeper shade for summer and a lighter shade for winter. Your skin can also have different needs in the summer versus winter: your skin may be oily in the summer and dry during the winter. So, be open to the idea that you might need a different foundation (shade and/or formula) for each season.

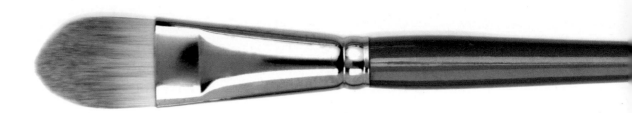

what type of finish do you want your foundation to provide?

There are basically four types of finishes you can achieve with foundation. Some work better than others for certain skin types.

matte is a great choice for almost every type of skin, from normal all the way to oily. The only exception is severely dry skin, because a matte finish can cause it to look even drier—and, in turn, older, rather than younger. A matte finish works best for skin with imperfections, such as breakouts, scars, and discoloration. (The more matte the skin, the more flawless it appears, because shine just accentuates textural flaws.) A matte finish provides the best coverage and is perfect for oily skin, because it contains no oils and won't increase the shine. Use a light hand, however, because applying it too heavily can make it appear mask-like.

dewy works well on dry skin because it adds moisture. It is wonderful for most skin types, except oily skin, where it can increase the shine and showcase flaws such as surface bumps and blemishes. Dewy foundation is not the best choice during summer or in high-humidity areas, because it can appear too shiny or greasy, instead of just dewy.

satin is a good choice for most skin types, with the exception of excessively oily skin. It gives the skin a soft, smooth appearance. This finish is extremely kind to skin texture (it's always true that the smoother the skin, the more youthful it appears). The finish is not as flat as matte, which has no sheen at all, nor as shiny as dewy, but falls between the two. Satin is the most common foundation finish and is perfect for making the skin look young and fresh.

luminous works well on almost all skin types. Its light-reflecting properties help hide tiny flaws and lines by reflecting light off the surface of the face, so it disguises imperfections. It is also great for giving the skin a youthful, healthy glow. But I would steer clear of this formula if you have oily skin, because it can make your face look shiny and greasy.

tip:

If you're buying foundation in a drugstore and can't try it out on your skin first, steer clear of shades that look pink in the bottle (they make your skin look unnaturally red, which ages the look of your skin). The slightest hint of yellow in a foundation, while not as appealing in the bottle, is actually much more universally flattering. It will help neutralize any red discoloration your skin may have.

> "the best tool
> is the tool you
> work best with"

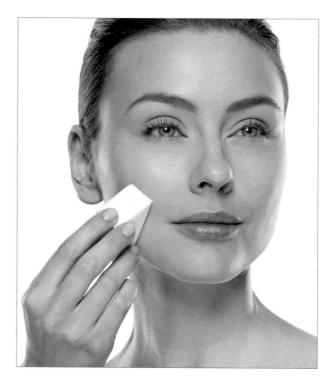

applying foundation

For applying foundation, you have three basic tools from which to choose. All three can provide great application, but I believe the best tool for you is the one you work best with. I could tell you a brush is the only way to go, but if you can't control a brush, you won't get the best application from it. The best tool is the tool you work best with.

Why does it matter? The better the application, the more flawless the skin will look. And the more flawless the skin, the younger you will look. Have I made my point?

• A sponge is the most sanitary, because I think you are more likely to wash it or throw it away after using it. You *must* clean it after every use, because there is no way to get perfect application from a sponge loaded with dried-up foundation from two days ago. The cleaner the tool, the better the application. Sponges also help with the blending process. I love sponges—I can really get the foundation and skin to look like one with them, because they blend so well.

You can control your coverage by using the sponge damp or dry and by stippling or wiping. A dry sponge provides more coverage, while a damp sponge makes your foundation go on sheerer. Stippling (a patting motion) gives more coverage; using your sponge to glide foundation across your face provides less coverage. You are in control! The better the sponge quality, the more flawless the application. With sponges, as with so many things, price does matter.

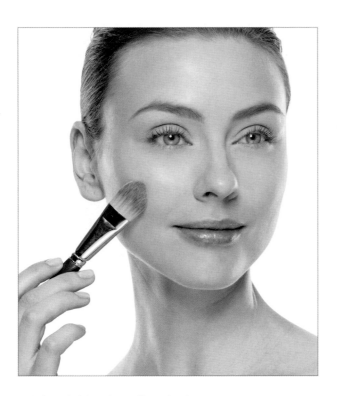

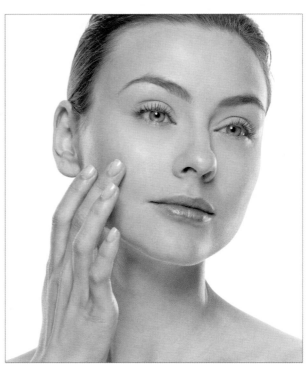

• A brush blends well, so it gives you great coverage. The head of a foundation brush is tapered to promote smooth, even coverage, helping your foundation to blend as you apply it. It is also great for those who want a little extra coverage, because a brush makes it really easy to achieve a fuller-coverage finish. It's also excellent for touching up the foundation you've worn all day. If you want to go out that evening, but you don't want to cleanse your face and start over, you can use the brush to apply more foundation over the product you have had on all day; it will go on flawlessly smooth. This is the one time a brush is the best choice, because it is the only tool that will not disturb the products you already have on your face. Like the sponge, your brush must be washed or cleansed after every application. (Repeat after me: The cleaner the tool, the better the application.) Foundation brushes are made of synthetic fibers, so they wash more easily and dry faster than natural-bristle brushes.

• Don't have a brush or sponge handy? No problem, because the third tool is your fingertips. Be sure to wash your hands after you've applied your moisturizer and treatment products and before you apply your foundation; the residue from the treatment products can compromise the integrity of your foundation and diminish the amount of coverage it provides. Your fingers can give beautiful, smooth coverage. But fingers are my least-favorite tool, only because I feel you get a better blend of your foundation with a sponge or a brush. But if this is the tool that works best for you, then your fingers are *your* perfect application tool.

stephanie, 30s

Stephanie's hooded eyelids draw attention away from her gorgeous eyes. The glow I gave her really makes her look her best. Narrowing her nose also made such a difference.

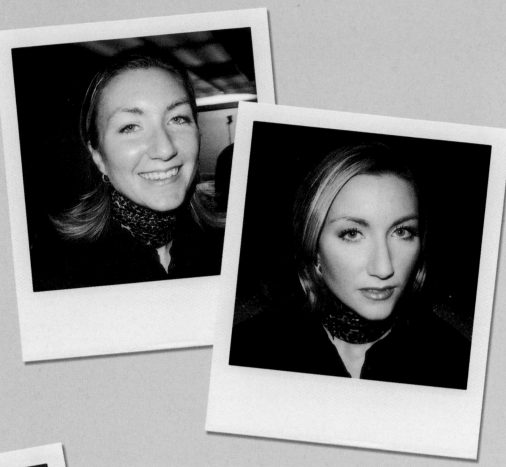

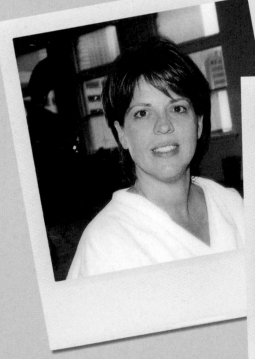

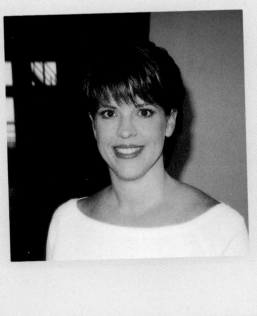

lisa, 40s

I had to lift Lisa's eyes. Droopy eyes immediately aged her. I loved that I was able to visually lift them. Eye makeup took years off— she's younger looking, definitely.

application basics

Whether you use a sponge, a brush, or your fingers, the best technique for applying foundation is to begin your application at the center of your face and work your way outward. You can dip your tool in foundation and apply it directly to the skin, or you can start by dotting foundation on the cheeks, the forehead, the chin, and the nose, then blend it outward. Always remember to finish with your final strokes blending downward (no matter what your tool choice), to make sure all the small facial hairs lie flat.

After application, give the foundation a couple of seconds to dry, then blot with a tissue to absorb any excess moisture left from the product. This simple blotting step can really enhance the staying power of your foundation. Be sure to finish with a light dusting of powder. If your skin is really dry, you do not have to powder your entire face: just dust your t-zone (center of forehead, nose, cheeks, and tip of the chin). I find that many women with dry skin still need to powder their t-zone, due to shine.

Applying your foundation properly is important for looking younger. As I've said over and over, the more flawless your skin looks, the younger *you* look. Experiment with multiple application tools until you find the one that does the best job for you. Every day is a new opportunity to look younger, because each day you have a chance to apply your makeup better than the day before.

tips:

Want your foundation to look as natural as possible? The best way to achieve a natural look is to first apply a sheer layer of foundation all over the face, then apply either another layer of foundation or concealer on any small imperfections.

Foundation isn't just for the skin. You can also apply it to your lips. Why do that, you ask? This technique creates a blank canvas for reshaping your lip line. It's also useful as an anchor for lipstick, because the foundation can help it stay on longer.

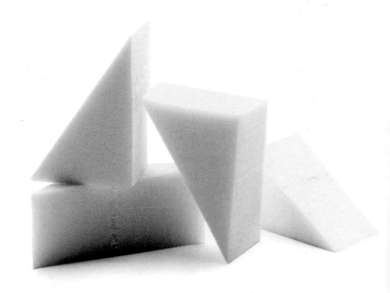

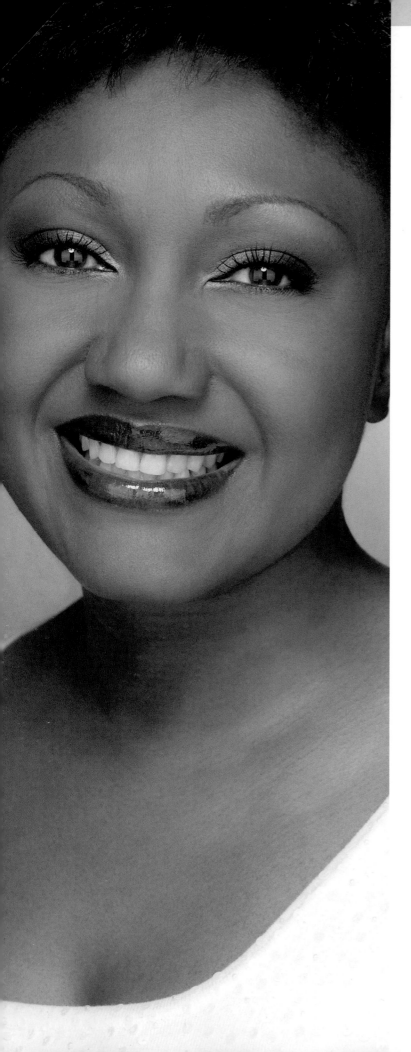

facial masking

Facial masking is a condition that can affect women with bronze/ebony skin tones. If your skin has a natural "mask"—that is, a tendency to be darker around the outer edges of the face and lighter in the interior of the face—you have facial masking. Probably one of the most important things to remember here is that it will take two shades of foundation to correct this.

Correcting facial masking is different from concealing other facial discolorations, because you are dealing with three shades of skin. One is the light area in the center of your face, the second is the darker area around the perimeter of your face (forehead, jawline, and around the mouth), and last, but certainly not least, is your neck and body, which are usually a different shade than the other two—generally lighter than the outer edges of your face, but darker than the center. It's worth the effort to correct this condition, though, because, as in every case, the more even and flawless your skin appears, the younger you will look.

With a little practice, it's easy to correct facial masking by using the following simple application techniques.

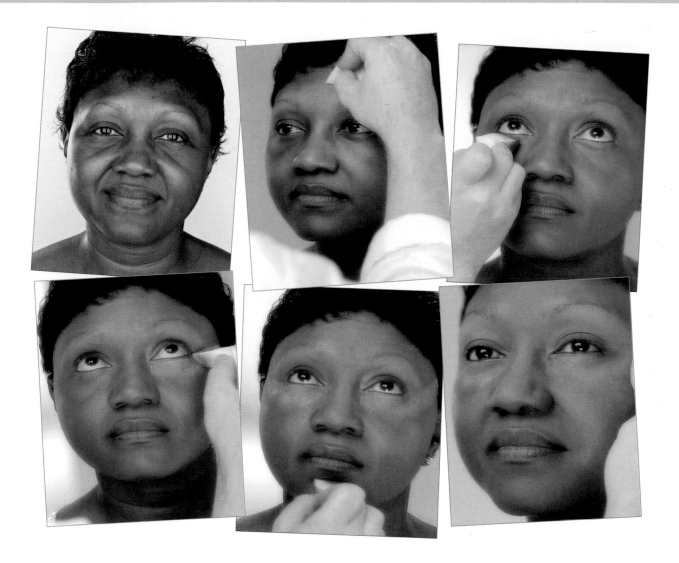

1. First, it's essential to conduct a stripe test from your cheek down to your jaw, to determine the two foundation shades you will need to create a more even complexion. See page 88 to learn how to do a stripe test. You'll need two foundation shades to correct your facial masking: one to brighten the darker areas and one to deepen the lighter areas. There is no way to fix this with one shade, because no single shade can lighten the darker area to match the lighter area and also not deepen the lighter area to match the dark (plus, you wouldn't want it to try this, because the darker area is darker than your neck and body). The goal of your stripe test is to find the two shades that, when applied to the opposite areas of your skin, meet in between (or make each area match the other) and provide a more even skin tone.

2. Apply the lighter shade of foundation just to the darker areas on your face.

3. Apply the darker shade of foundation only to the lighter areas on your face. Applying the correct shade of foundation to the appropriate shade of skin will correct your skin tones and make your skin look even and flawless.

4. Once your skin tone has been evened out, you can determine the shade of powder you need— you have to see what color your skin becomes before you can know what shade of powder to use. For example, if you were to choose the shade that matched the darkest foundation, it would make your face too dark. Now that you can see what shade of powder you need, apply powder to set your makeup.

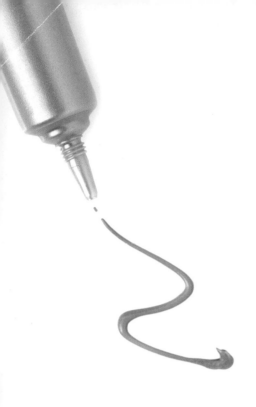

concealer

What can age you the most is uneven, discolored skin. Because of this, concealer can be your best friend, because it can improve your skin's appearance dramatically—but only if it's invisible. The secret to concealing what you don't want to see is applying concealer just to the discolored skin. Learn to color within the lines, just like when you learned to color as a child!

You must be careful with concealer, however, because it has a different texture than foundation (drier and thicker, because it is designed to stick, and that is what it does) Because of this, it can draw attention to fine lines if you are not careful when applying it, especially if you use too much. As a result, it is imperative that you choose the right formula for the job. If you use a formula that is too moist, it can "travel," slipping into creases and fine lines, drawing attention to your flaws. A formula that is too dry is bad for the delicate skin around the eyes and can draw attention to those flaws. Experiment to find the perfect formula for you. Consult the product knowledge chapter (Chapter 3, page 29) to find out which formula works best to conceal what you are trying to hide.

Once you've chosen the perfect concealer texture, you need to make the right color choice. Choose the same shade as your foundation, or a shade that is one shade lighter, for most things you want to conceal. For extremely dark discoloration, choose a shade that is two levels lighter than your foundation. Just be sure not to choose a shade that is too light, because it can end up looking grey and ashy.

You can get a lot of mileage out of concealers with yellow undertones. Yellow is the best color choice for severe discoloration of ivory/beige skin, because it works to counteract the colors of most skin imperfections, including the purple of under-eye circles, the brown of age spots, and any ruddiness or red in your complexion. The more severe the imperfection—such as a port-wine stain or extremely dark circles—the more yellow you will want in your concealer.

tip:

If the discoloration is only slight, try covering it with a second layer of foundation, before you break out the concealer. You can also use a second foundation that gives more coverage for just such a circumstance (try a stick foundation, it's great for this) and apply it just to the areas that need the extra coverage.

"a big part of looking younger is taking the right steps and making the right choices to achieve your goals"

For bronze/ebony skin, a golden orange concealer for light to medium skin tones works wonderfully. For really deep tones of ebony, a warm brown concealer usually covers best. Again, the more intense the skin discoloration, the more intense the concealer undertone color should be, so that it can be more corrective.

If you're using a concealer that matches your foundation exactly, you can apply it either before or after your foundation. If you're using one that is lighter than your foundation, it is best to apply it first.

Let's face it: Very few women have perfectly flawless skin. Yet many women are obsessed with perfection! Everything from sun damage to genetics can affect your complexion, especially as you get older. Fortunately, we can disguise most if not all of these imperfections. In the pages that follow, we will learn all the *looking younger* techniques needed to do just that.

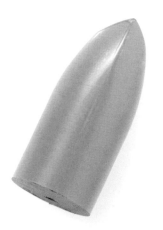

tips:

Using a concealer that's too light in depth can actually draw more attention to the flaws you are trying to cover.

Concealer can be made more sheer by mixing it with a little eye crème or moisturizer before you apply it.

You can test the coverage of a concealer by applying a little to a vein on the inside of your wrist.

When concealing, slowly building your coverage with multiple light layers looks the most natural. So, don't be heavy-handed! Use a light touch and just a little product on your brush, rather than a lot.

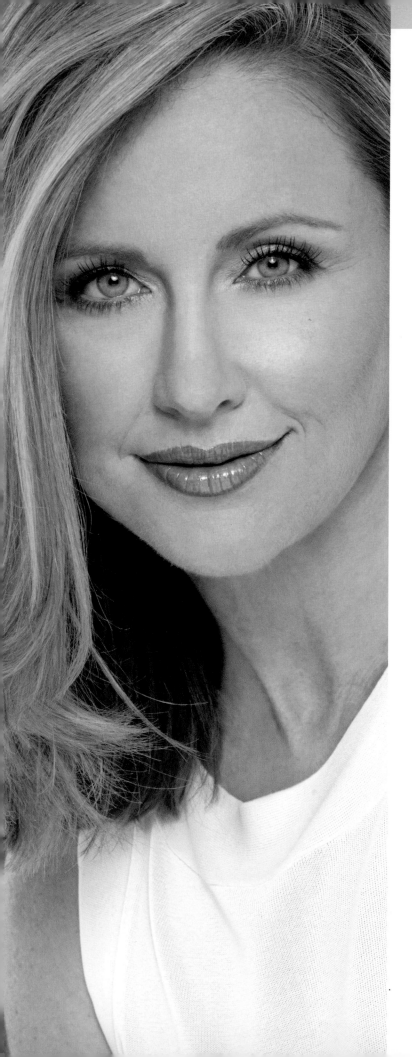

dark circles

Concealer can draw attention to fine lines, and the place we most often find those lines is around the eye. Skin in the under-eye area contains fewer oil glands than anywhere else on your body, so it needs plenty of moisture. The more moist and supple you make this area before you apply your concealer, the better the results. Keeping this in mind, let's go through covering dark circles step by step:

1. Prepare the area underneath the eye by applying eye crème and letting it soak in for a couple of minutes. If it is really dry, feel free to apply an extra layer and let it soak in and dry. Be generous with your eye crème, because it's next to impossible to over-moisturize this area. Just be sure to blot off any excess crème after a few minutes with a sponge or tissue, to make sure your concealer stays put. Using eye crème will help your concealer adhere and prevents it from caking up and drawing attention to fine lines, if the skin under your eyes tends to be dry.

2. Next, use a brush to apply concealer along the line of demarcation—where the discoloration begins on your skin. Extend the concealer up and over the entire discolored area with your brush (stay just slightly below your lower lash line, because applying your concealer right up to the lower lash line can close your eye in and make it look smaller). You never want to extend the concealer past the line of demarcation (onto the skin that you are tying to match). If you do, you will lighten skin that is already the correct color, and you'll be back where you started— with two uneven shades of skin.

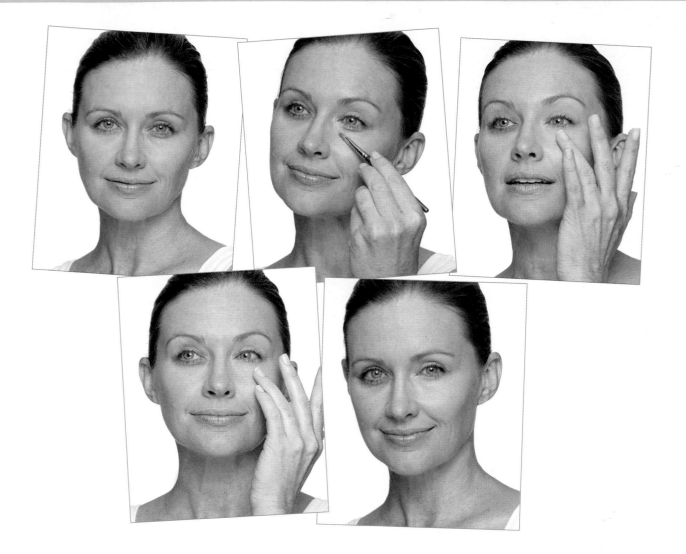

3. Now, with your finger, and using a stippling (patting) motion, stipple the concealer along the line of demarcation to blend it in. This blends in the texture of the concealer and helps to make it invisible. Be sure to conceal any darkness in the inside corners of your eyes or eyelids, if necessary.

4. When applying foundation over an area you have just concealed, be sure to stipple or pat it on. You don't want to wipe away what you just concealed.

5. Always finish with a light dusting of powder to set your handiwork.

Serious dark circles call for serious concealer. Use one that is a shade or two lighter than your foundation and apply the concealer before your foundation. Yellow concealers are a great choice for covering severe dark circles on ivory/beige skin, and golden orange concealers work well for bronze/ebony skin. These are called corrective concealers, because they counteract the look of severe discoloration. Both concealers can counteract all shades of skin discoloration, from red to purple to brown.

Q&A

Every time I use concealer under my eyes to cover some darkness, it just draws attention to my fine lines. Is there anything that I can do to prevent this?

First, you need to make sure to moisturize under your eye with an eye crème. This helps keep the skin supple and full of moisture, so that when you apply your concealer, it will draw less attention to fine lines. You can also make your concealer more moisturizing by mixing it with your eye crème before you apply it.

I have really deep, dark under-eye circles, so I use a very light shade of concealer to cover the darkness. But when I am finished, the area appears too light and ashy. How can I fix this?

This is completely understandable, because you need a lighter shade to cover the darkness. Even a wonderful corrective color like yellow can leave the under-eye area a little light and ashy looking, especially on darker beige skin tones. If you have just finished concealing and the area appears a little too light and ashy, no worries. To remedy this problem, simply dust a very light amount of a subtle bronzer (matte, not one with shimmer in it) over the area. It will warm it up just enough to cut the ashy, overly light appearance.

As I go through my day, the skin under my eyes starts to appear dry and crepey. What can I do?

You can add moisture back to this area without messing up your concealer. Actually, you can moisturize as frequently as you like. Lightly pat a tiny bit of eye crème over the area. Do not rub it or work it in, just pat it on. The crème you put on top will melt in. Be sure to leave it alone after you pat it on. This will rehydrate the area and get rid of the dry, crepey appearance.

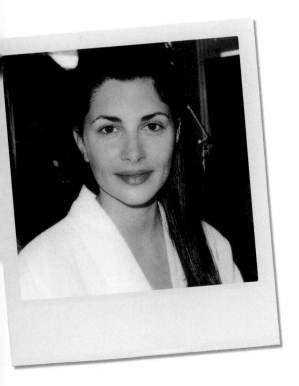

blemishes

It comes as a surprise to some people, but blemishes can strike at any age. To minimize the appearance of facial blemishes or pimples, use a concealer with a dry texture; it will cling to the blemish better, last throughout the day, and not irritate the skin or initiate more breakouts.

Here are the easy quick steps to perfection:

1. Apply your foundation first. This is definitely one instance in which you want to always apply your foundation before you conceal. It makes the process much easier.

2. Choose a concealer with a dry texture, being sure to choose one with a depth level that is not lighter than your foundation. Your concealer should match your skin exactly. A light concealer will only make the blemish seem larger, because everything we lighten comes forward. Using a brush, apply the concealer directly to the blemish.

3. With your finger, use a stippling (patting) motion to blend the edges around the blemish into the skin. Stippling blends in the texture of the concealer, making it invisible. For stubborn blemishes, feel free to apply a second layer for extra coverage.

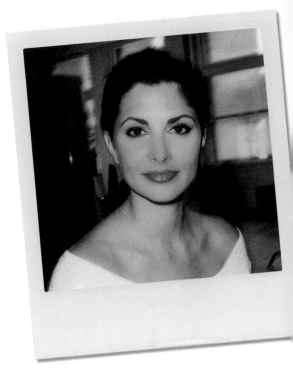

tips:

A great choice for covering blemishes (and anywhere you need precise application) is a concealer pencil. Its precision application and drier texture make it perfect for this purpose.

If you have a lot of redness around the area in which a blemish is rising (but no broken skin: you have not picked at it and it has not exploded), try this trick: Use a cotton swab and apply a little Visine directly to the area. It will calm the redness, making the blemish easier to cover.

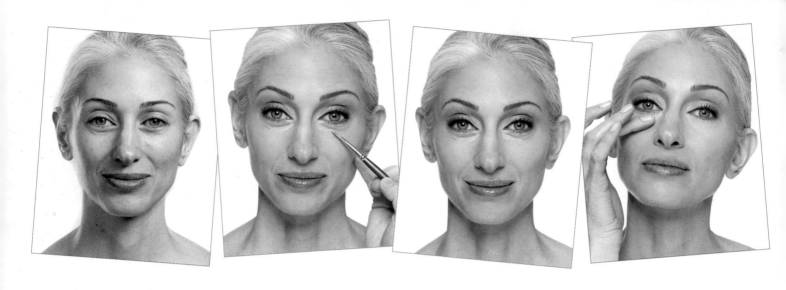

under-eye puffiness

Under-eye puffiness is when the area under the eye is raised and puffed. Because it is raised and stands out away from the skin, the fact that you are usually lit from above accentuates the puffiness, by creating a shadow underneath the puffy area. This draws even more attention to your problem. You cannot improve the appearance of under-eye puffiness by swiping a light concealer under the eye area, because anything we lighten just stands out even more. Our goal is to disguise the puffy area, not make it more prominent.

You can outsmart the puffiness by highlighting the shadowy area just underneath it. This helps to bring it out and make it appear even with the rest of the face, not indented. Because most people look directly at you and not from above, your puffiness will appear even with the rest of your skin. Voilà—you're flawless!

Use the following four quick steps to disguise under-eye puffiness.

1. First, apply your foundation. The process of disguising the puffiness starts after you apply your foundation.

2. Next, take a highlighting pen (for more info on this product, visit Chapter 3, page 29) and apply it just underneath the puffiness, right where the shadow is being created. Be sure not to extend the product up onto the puffy area, because it

will just make it look puffier. The highlighting pen has light-reflecting properties, which make the recessed area appear to come forward, so it's even with the rest of the face and we do not see the indented area.

3. Now use your finger to stipple (a patting motion) along the highlighted area. This will blend in the color and texture of the highlighter, making it invisible.

4. Lightly powder, and move on with your life.

If you have dark circles as well as puffiness, which some women do, you'll need to take one extra step in your application to achieve perfection:

1. Apply concealer to your dark circles first, following the application method on page 106. Be sure to apply it only to the discolored skin and then stipple the edges to blend.

2. Next, apply your foundation.

3. Now, apply the highlighting pen right underneath the puffiness, where the shadow is being created (as in the previous Step 2).

4. Use your finger to stipple along the highlighted area, to blend in the color and texture of your highlighter, making it invisible.

5. Lightly powder, and you're done.

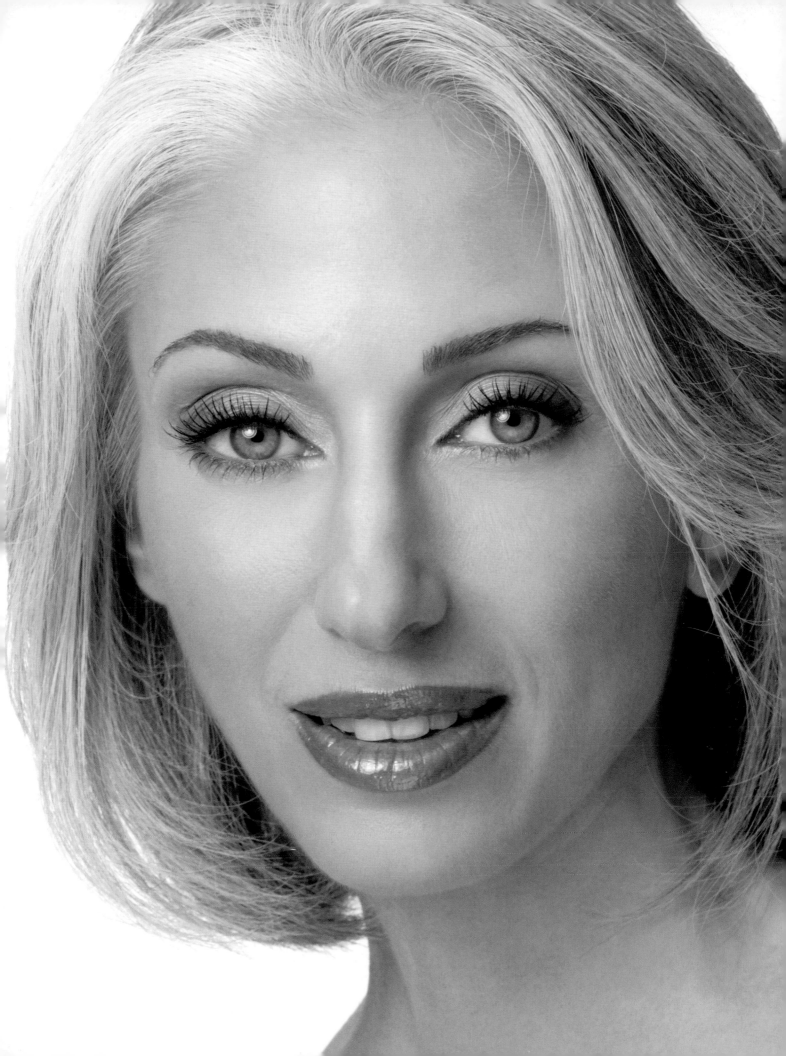

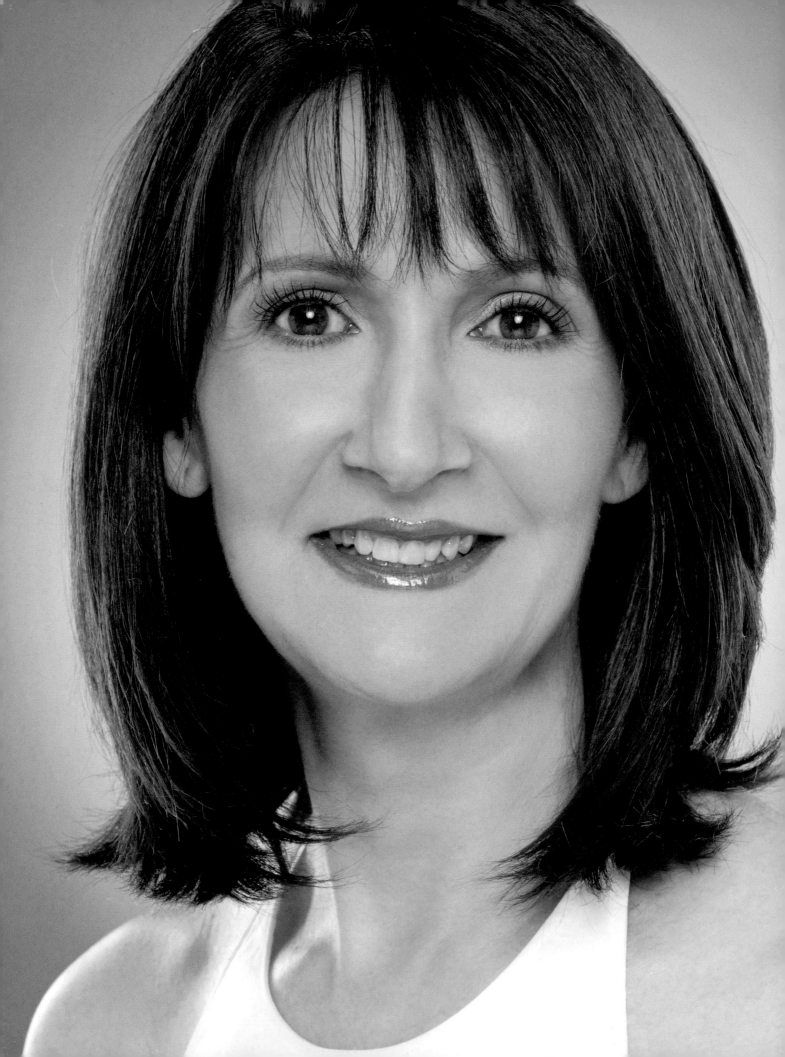

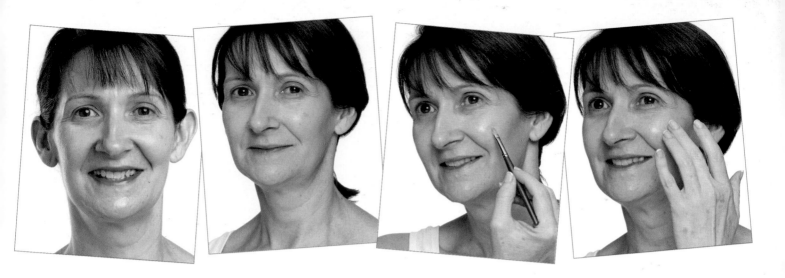

hyperpigmentation and melasma

Hyperpigmentation is a common condition in which patches of skin become darker in color than the normal surrounding skin. This darkening occurs when an excess of melanin, the brown pigment that produces normal skin color, forms deposits in the skin. Hyperpigmentation can affect women of every skin tone. Age spots are a common form of hyperpigmentation. They occur due to sun damage. Many women develop them after they start having hot flashes, as age spots are also caused by a shift in hormones during menopause. These small, darkened patches are usually found on the hands, face, and other areas frequently exposed to the sun.

Melasma (chloasma) spots are similar in appearance to age spots but are larger areas of darkened skin that appear most often as a result of hormonal changes. Pregnancy, for example, can trigger an overproduction of melanin that causes "pregnancy masking" on the face.

If you are prone to hyperpigmentation, *stay out of the sun* (sun exposure just increases the problem) and wear lots of sun block. Whether you have one large spot (more common with pregnancy masking) or multiple small spots, you must cover each spot individually, applying concealer only to the discolored areas. If you extend the concealer past the line of demarcation, you will lighten skin that is already the correct color and re-create multiple shades of skin.

Here are the steps to follow:

1. Using a brush for precision (unless you have a very large spot—then you can use your fingers or a sponge), apply your concealer only to the dark, discolored area (color within the lines). If the discoloration is severe (very brown), women with ivory/beige skin tones should use a yellow pigmented concealer (the yellow will neutralize the brown in the spots). Women with bronze/ebony skin tones should use a concealer with a golden orange undertone, to help neutralize the dark brown color of the spot. If there are multiple spots, cover each one separately.

2. Using your finger, stipple (a patting motion) around the outer edges of every concealed spot. This will blend in the texture, making the area look completely natural.

3. Now apply your foundation, being sure to stipple it over the concealed areas. Stippling prevents the concealer from being removed. If you were to wipe your foundation over these areas, you could remove the concealer.

4. Finish with a light dusting of powder, to set everything and make it last throughout the day.

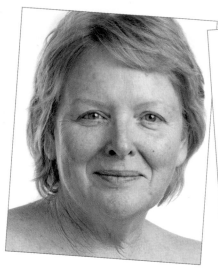
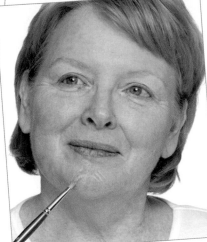
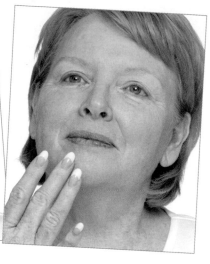

broken capillaries or veins

As with hyperpigmentation, when covering broken capillaries or veins, it is important to apply concealer only to the discolored areas. Color within the lines. This can be a little harder with broken capillaries or veins, because we have to be so exact.

Step by step, here's what to do:

1. Use a brush to draw a line of concealer along the broken capillary or vein. Don't try to cover the general area; you must apply it only to the vein. Extending the concealer past the edges of the vein or broken capillary only lightens the skin you are trying to match, disguising nothing. This is why a concealer brush makes everything so much easier—it's precise. Also, using a concealer pencil for concealing veins is amazing—you simply draw it right along the vein (it could not be any easier).

2. Now, using the tip of your finger, stipple along the concealed lines, to blend in the texture of your concealer and make it look completely natural.

3. Next, apply your foundation. Remember to stipple (a patting motion) your foundation over the area when you're applying it over an area already concealed.

4. Finish by powdering, to set your makeup and help it last all day.

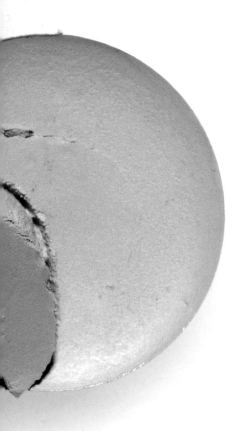

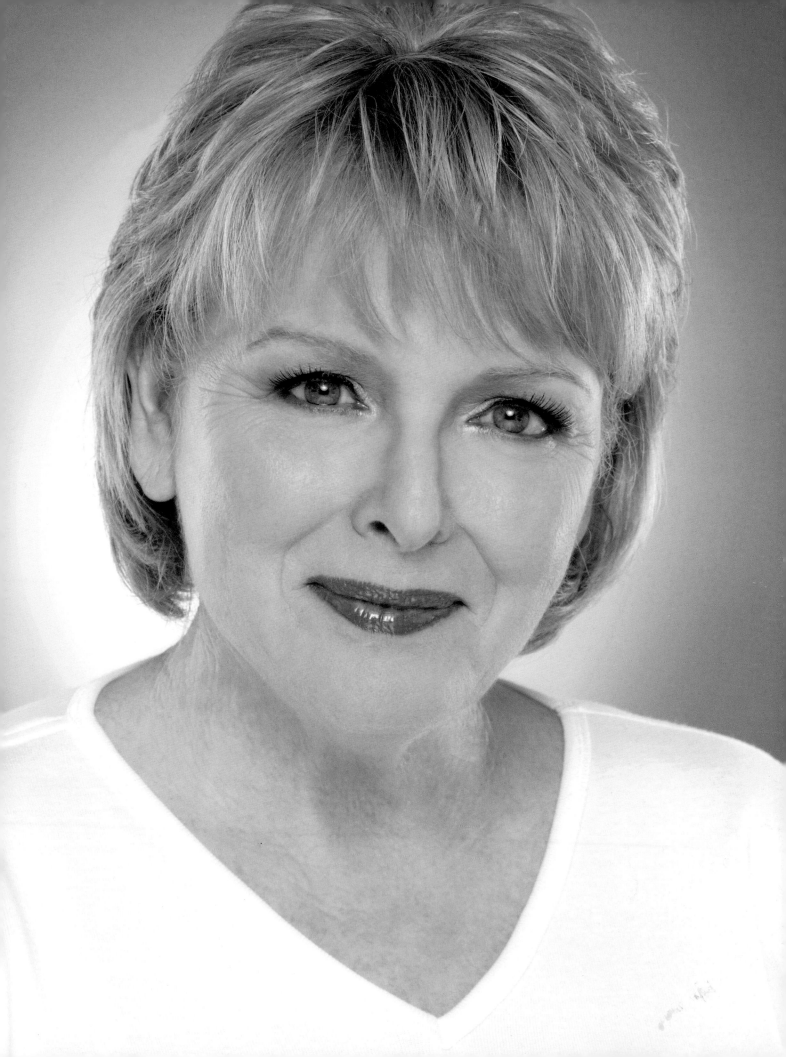

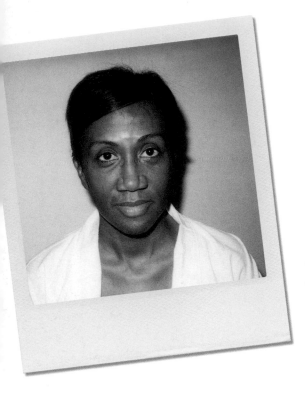

rosacea

Rosacea is an area of redness on the skin. It most commonly occurs in the cheek area and across the nose, as well as the chin and sometimes the forehead. A lot of women develop slight cases of rosacea after they start having "their own private summers," due to the hormonal changes of menopause. Some women have rosacea their whole lives.

Rosacea usually appears as a general area of redness, marked with darker red spots. I prefer to use as little concealer as possible when disguising imperfections, so I conceal rosacea using a few extra steps:

1. To counteract the redness of rosacea, use a yellow-based concealer. Apply a thin layer of concealer to all the red areas. Although this thin layer will cover the general area of redness, probably a few darker areas of redness will still show through. No problem—we will tackle these next.

2. Using the same concealer, apply another layer to the darker areas —but only to the spots that are still visible. By covering in two steps, you will avoid having a thick layer of concealer over a large area of your face, and your skin will look more natural.

3. Stipple (a patting motion) around the outer edges of the concealed area, to blend in the texture.

4. Apply your foundation now, but be sure to stipple, not wipe, your foundation over the concealed areas. Wiping on your foundation can remove the product from the area you just concealed.

5. Finish with a light dusting of powder.

Most women do not want to wear blush after they have concealed their rosacea. After all, they just covered the excess color in their cheeks — the last thing they want to do is add color back to this area. If you do want some color back in your cheeks, choose something very natural. A great option is to use a little bronzer for color, rather than blush.

vitiligo or hypopigmentation

Vitiligo (also called hypopigmentation and leukoderma) is a chronic skin condition that causes loss of pigment, resulting in irregular patches of pale skin. With vitiligo, we are still dealing with spots, but instead of dark spots, these are light spots. We still have to color within the lines when applying concealer to light spots, because extending the concealer past the line of demarcation creates multiple shades of skin.

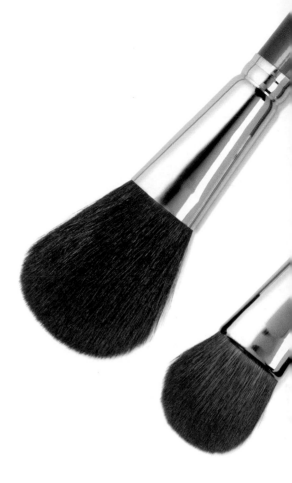

Concealing a vitiligo spot differs from our previous methods in that, instead of using a concealer to lighten a spot, we actually need one to darken it. Your natural skin tone determines the level of contrast between your concealer choice and your skin. For example, the deeper your skin tone, the deeper the concealer shade you will need. If you have beige skin, you will probably need a shade of concealer only one to two levels darker than your natural skin. But if you have bronze/ebony skin, you will probably need a shade two to three levels darker than your natural skin tone, because the contrast of depth between the spot and your skin is much more dramatic.

The steps for concealing unpigmented spots are the same as those for concealing dark spots, except that we use a darker concealer. Here are the quick and easy steps to a flawless face:

1. Using a brush for precision (unless it is a very large spot, in which case you can use your fingers or a sponge), apply your concealer only to the light, discolored area. If there are multiple spots, cover each one separately.

2. Using your finger, stipple (a patting motion) around the outer edges of every spot that you concealed. This will blend in the texture, making the skin look completely natural.

3. Now, apply your foundation, being sure to stipple it over the concealed areas, to avoid inadvertently removing the concealer.

4. Finish with a light dusting of powder, to set your makeup and help it last throughout the day.

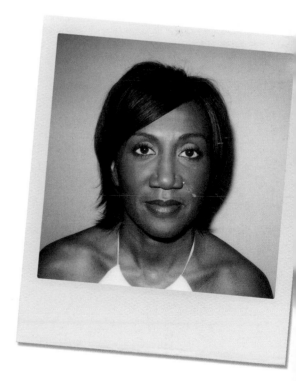

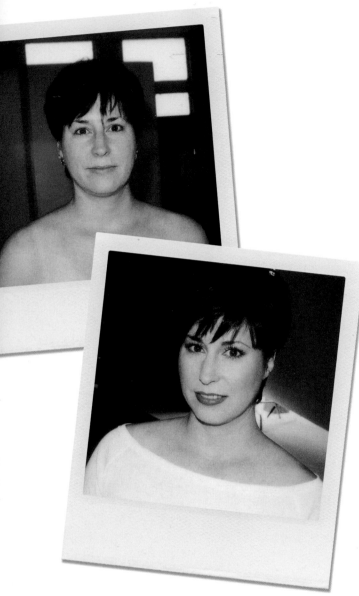

rhonda, 40s

Rhonda has gorgeous skin, but she needed a bit of color. I had to draw attention to those beautiful eyes.

scars

Scars are especially tricky to conceal, because a scar is an area of skin without pores, and pores are what makeup clings to on the skin. I am sure many of you have had the experience of trying to cover a scar and finding that no product seems to stick or adhere to the area. You try to apply foundation, and it just slips right off. To get concealer to adhere to a scar, you will need one with a much drier texture than one you would use under your eyes. If you do not want to invest in multiple concealers, you can adjust your normal concealer, so that it will adhere to the scar.

If your concealer has a dry texture and is designed to conceal scars, a few easy steps are all that are required for flawless, younger-looking skin:

1. With a concealer brush, apply your concealer directly to the scar (and only to the scar).
2. Use your finger to stipple (a patting motion) around and along the edges of the concealed area, to blend in the texture of your concealer and make it invisible.
3. Now, apply your foundation, being sure to stipple the foundation over your scar. Do not wipe it on — you don't want to expose the scar you have just concealed.
4. Lightly powder, to set your makeup and make it last all day.

If you want to use the same concealer that you use under your eyes, you just need to add a couple of extra steps to adjust its texture and help it stick:

1. Lightly moisturize the scarred area.
2. Powder the scar with a tiny bit of loose powder. The moisturizer gives the powder something to cling to and helps it adhere to the scarred area..

3. With a concealer brush, apply your concealer directly to the scar (and only to the scar). The concealer and powder will mix together, creating a drier texture that will adhere to the scar.

4. Next, use your finger to stipple around and along the edges of the concealed area, to blend in the texture of your concealer and make it invisible.

5. Now, apply your foundation, being sure to stipple the foundation over your scar. Do not wipe it on—you don't want to remove the concealer-powder blend.

6. Finish by lightly powdering, to set your makeup and help it last all day.

For acne scars, which create texture variation in your skin, the best way to make the skin look perfectly flawless is to keep it as matte as possible. Loose powder is your best friend, because it will do just that. You want to be sure to keep the oil and shine away all day, so blot often, and use loose powder to matte the skin.

Keep the finish of the color products you choose in mind, as well. Avoid using products that add shimmer to your skin. For example, if you use bronzer (which I believe you should, always), it needs to be matte, with no sparkle or shimmer at all. The same is true for your blush; use a matte shade, not one with shimmer. The sparkle or shimmer in these products makes the skin look shiny, which will accentuate your textural flaws. The more matte the skin, the more flawless it will appear.

Finally, resist the temptation to fill in the "valleys" by applying too much foundation and concealer. Trying to cover up the textural flaws with thick, heavy layers of concealer and foundation just makes your skin look old and caked. A nice, smooth matte layer will make you look younger and fresher, and will make your skin appear flawless.

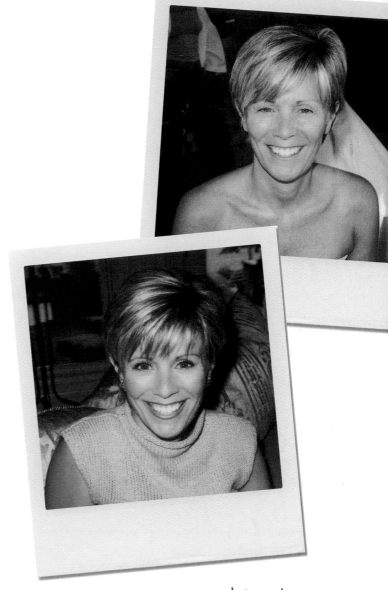

debi, 40s

I needed to make Debi's lips look fuller. The right technique and the right color helped achieve my goal. Fuller lips always look younger.

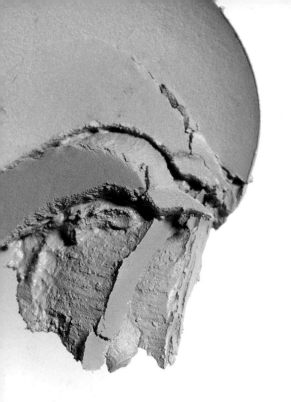

last thoughts about concealer

One last point I need to discuss with you is something that most women do not know. Concealers are very different from foundations. They are drier, more heavily pigmented, and they "grab" powder differently. Because of this, you have to be careful when you powder over a concealer. It is best to use a lighter shade of powder on a heavily concealed area. If you use the same shade of powder used for the rest of your face, the concealed area will grab the powder and appear darker.

I am sure many of you have experienced that proud moment when you concealed a dark spot on your cheek. You used your concealer brush to apply your concealer just to the discolored skin, then you stippled around the edges to blend it in. You looked in the mirror, and voila! No spot. Next, you applied your foundation, stippling it over the concealed area, to avoid removing the concealer. You are so proud of your flawless skin. You are a pro! Then you powder to set everything, and suddenly the spot is back. What happened? The concealer (because of its texture) grabbed the powder that matched your foundation (and your face) and turned darker. Using a powder that is a shade or two lighter, just on the concealed area, will prevent this from happening.

tips:

Yellow-based concealer shades look healthier and more natural, making the skin look youthful.

Using corrective green, pink, or violet concealers on ivory/beige skin will only turn your face colors. Yellow will counteract every discoloration and it will look more natural, because all of us have some yellow in our skin.

To get that perfect shade of concealer, try mixing it with a little of your foundation. This way, you can achieve an exact match.

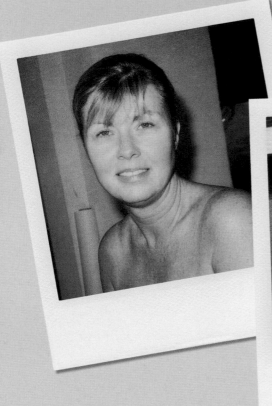

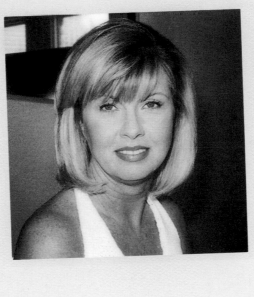

julie, 50s

All I could see was the fact that none of Julie's features really popped. I love the way I was able to draw attention to her beautiful lips and her eyes.

kathy, 40s

Kathy's face is so much lighter than her body. Thankfully, she is protecting her face from the sun. Making her face match her body really brought her natural beauty into focus and gave her skin the perfect glow.

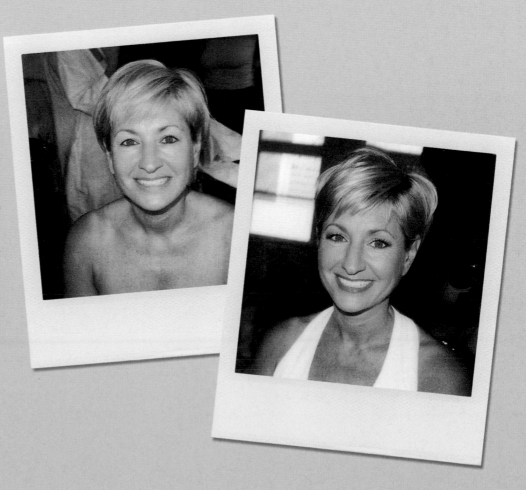

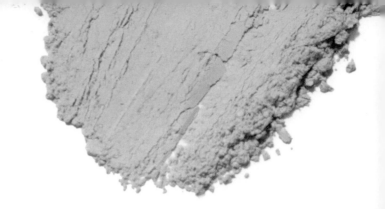

powder

Powder is a makeup must. It sets your foundation (and anything you have concealed), polishes your look, and adds a smooth, velvety softness to the skin. Because loose powder contains more oil absorbers than pressed powder, I prefer to use it to set the foundation. I then use pressed powder for touch-ups throughout the day, because it is quick and easy to carry.

When choosing a shade of powder, select one that matches your foundation; the powder will reinforce everything you have applied (foundation, concealer, highlighting pen) rather than fight it. Another option is to use a translucent powder, which is fine for paler skin tones, but remember that translucent does not mean the powder has no color. Translucent powder is not invisible (transparent), although the two words are easy to confuse. It is less opaque than other powders, but it is not colorless, and it can often appear unnatural and ashy on dark beige, olive, bronze, and ebony skin tones. Using a powder that is too light makes your skin look older. Translucent powder *is* helpful when powdering heavily concealed areas on ivory/beige skin (but never bronze/ebony skin).

There are several ways to apply powder:

- A brush is the easiest and most commonly used tool. It provides the lightest powder coverage. It is great for blending, but you must be careful not to over-blend and brush off what you apply. For best results, use a brush to apply a little powder at a time to ensure smooth, even coverage. If you are using loose powder, simply dip your brush in the powder, then tap it in the palm of your hand (or the top of the powder jar) to remove the excess. Apply what's left on the brush to your face. Then,

use your brush to pick up the powder that's left in your palm and finish applying it to your face.

- A powder puff offers the best coverage and is my favorite way to apply powder. Press your puff into the powder, tap the excess off in the palm of your hand, and then "roll" what is left on the puff onto your skin. Now grab the leftover powder in your palm with the puff and finish applying it to your face. Pushing it into the skin makes your foundation, powder and skin appear as one and look completely natural. To finish, lightly sweep your face with a brush, using gentle, downward strokes to remove any excess powder.

- A fingertip works well for a light powder application. It's a great way to powder underneath the eyes, especially for mature women. Dip your finger in loose powder. Rub your finger in the palm of your hand to brush off the excess, then trace your finger over the area underneath the eyes, to set your concealer and help minimize your chance of drawing attention to fine lines.

- A sponge works well for tight areas and is great for "spot" powdering

Q&A **I have very dry skin. Do I still need to powder my face after applying foundation and concealer?**

Absolutely! You may not need to powder your whole face because of your dry skin, but I find that even women with dry skin need to powder their t-zone area (center of face, forehead, nose, front of the cheeks, and tip of the chin) to cut the shine.

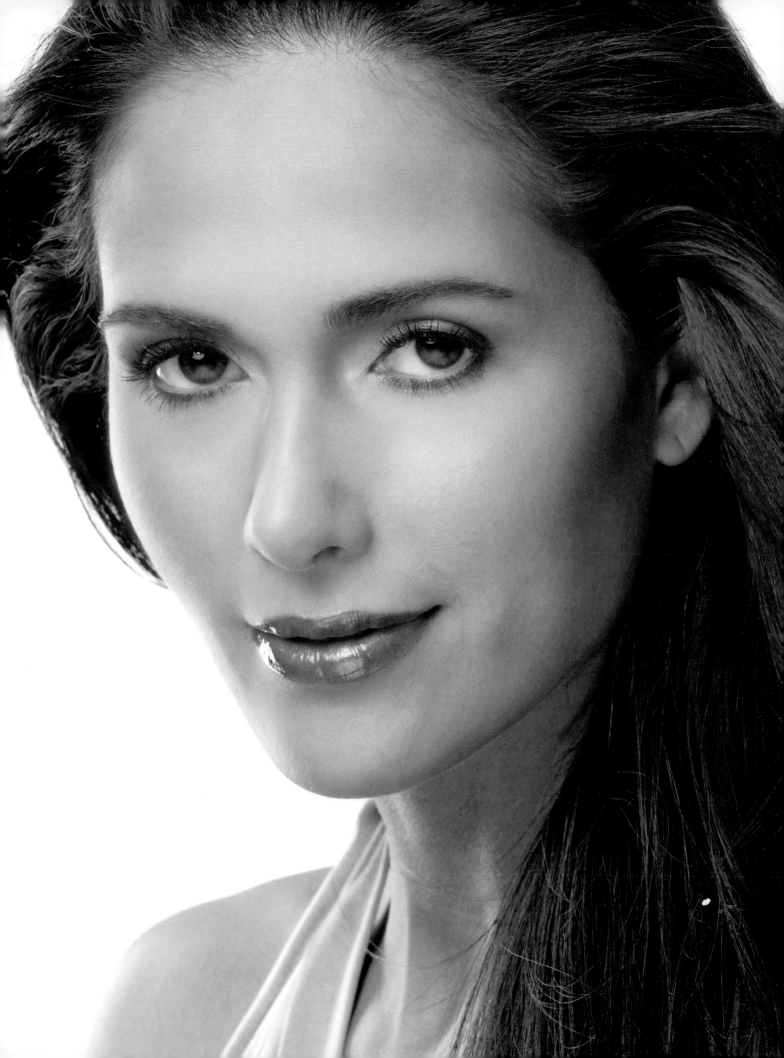

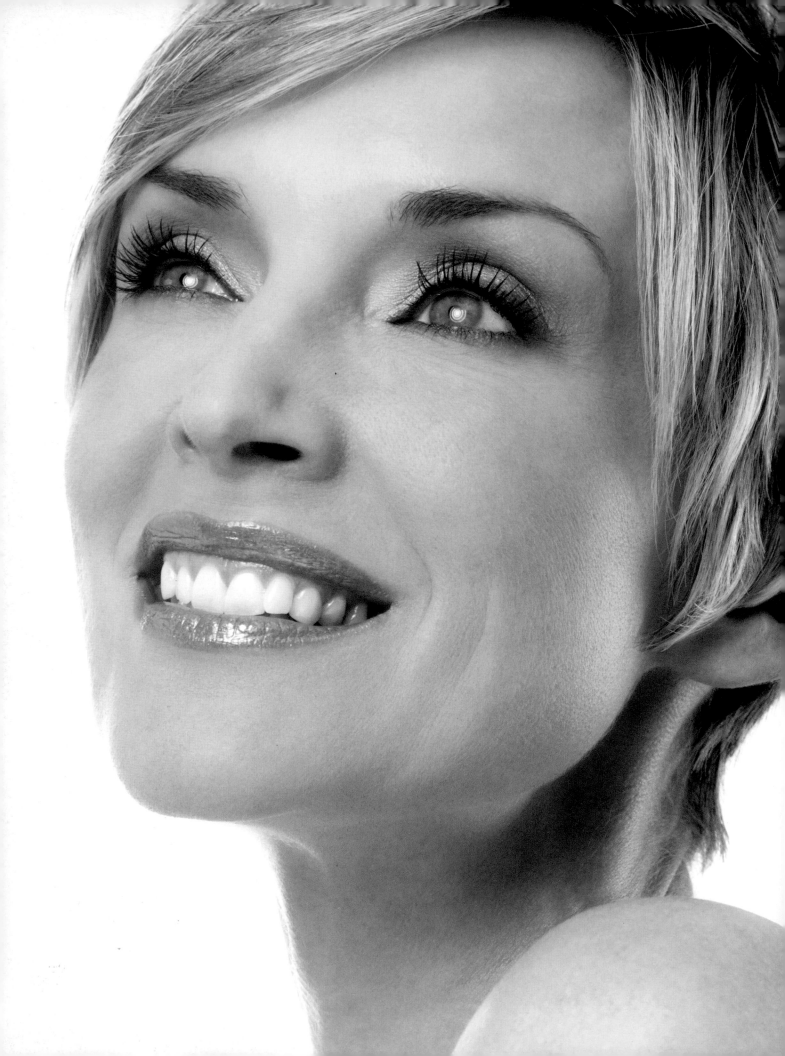

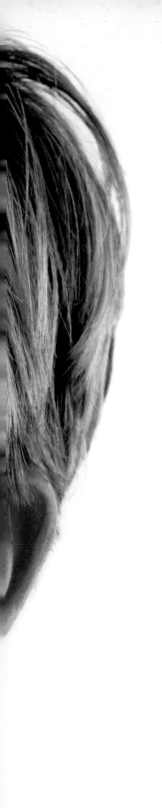

7

look 5 years younger and 5 pounds thinner

One of the biggest drawbacks to aging is that you lose pigment and color in your skin as you age, making you look pale and washed out. That is why making your skin appear lighter than its natural tone makes you look older. I can't count the number of times women have asked me how to add color and life to their face to help them look younger. Of course, one of the best ways is with a warmer, brighter, more colorful blush and lipstick, but we will get into that in later chapters.

A perfect way to add color to your face is by "sculpting the face"—blending multiple shades of foundation and powder in specific areas. The beauty of this technique is that it adds depth to the skin and shape to the face but looks completely natural. Adding dimension and color to your face will definitely give you that youthful glow you have been looking for.

How many of you have looked in the mirror and thought your face looked too full? Many women believe their face is too full (they think fat—not usually the case) and want to make it look slimmer. Believe it or not, it's simple to do. Keep in mind that you are just creating a subtle change, not performing surgery! By sculpting the face, you can slim down its appearance by using dark and light shades to subtly reshape it.

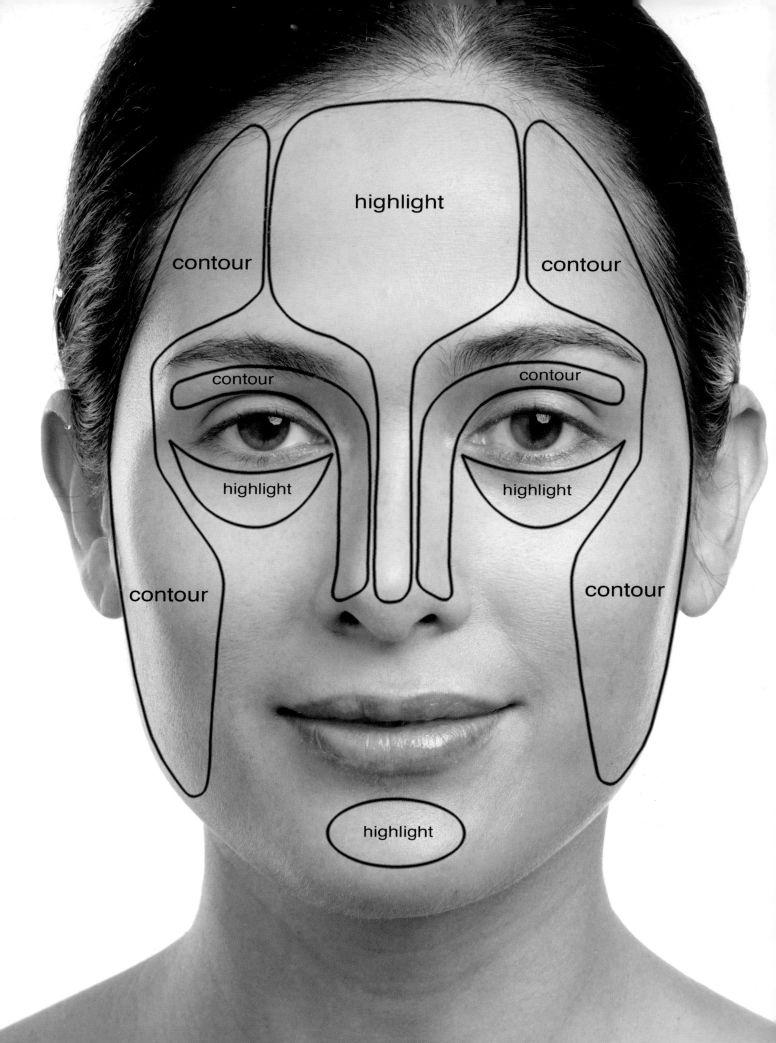

sculpting the face

The perfect face shape is considered to be oval, and your goal in sculpting your face is to make it appear more oval-shaped. You can make any face look more oval with nothing more exotic than foundation and powder. You will be surprised at the way this subtle effect can add the most incredible youthful glow to your skin.

The basic "sculpting" method involves highlighting and contouring your face. Think of it this way: Everything you highlight (or lighten) comes forward, and everything you contour (or darken) recedes. By sculpting your face, you pull forward the areas of your face we want to see (the oval area) and push back the areas you do not want to see. Minimizing the fullness around the outer edges of your face makes your face look slimmer, gives you a beautiful, youthful glow and adds color and depth to the skin.

Before you start, you will need to select three shades of foundation or powder in three different depth levels.

1. The first shade should match your skin exactly. It is your true foundation color. Visit Chapter 6 (page 87), to learn how to find your perfect shade.

2. The second color, your highlight color, should be one level lighter than the first, preferably with the same undertone.

3. The third shade, your contour color, should be one level darker than your first, preferably with the same undertone.

If you want your final result to be more dramatic, use three shades with more contrast between the depth levels. For example, if you want your contouring to be more noticeable and dramatic, use a shade two to three levels darker than your natural shade. To create contrast and more impact for ebony skin, choose a highlight shade two to three levels lighter than your natural shade. Keep in mind, however, that the more dramatic your choices, the more thoroughly and carefully you will need to blend the shades together.

The diagram on the left will help you understand the purpose and placement of your three shades. You can also refer to the face-shape diagrams starting on page 131 in this chapter, which provide customized application diagrams for a variety of face shapes. Be sure to blend the three shades really well, because it is the blending process that makes the sculpting method work and look natural.

tip:

Do you hate the appearance of your nose? Do you think it looks too wide? Here's an easy trick for narrowing its appearance. Highlight down the center of your nose the width that you want your nose to appear. Then place your contour shade along the sides of your nose, starting from your highlight shade and wrapping around and down the sides. This will make your nose appear narrower, because the eye will be drawn to the high-lighted area.

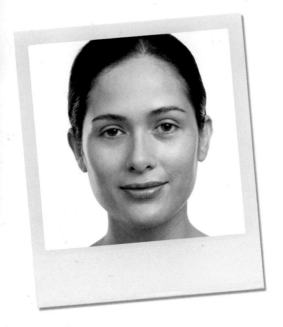

1. Apply your first, or true, foundation color over your entire face. Then visualize an oval on your face. The width of the oval is your eye sockets; the height and length of your oval extends from the tip of your forehead to the tip of your chin. Visualizing an oval helps you to see where to highlight and where to contour.

2. Apply your second, or highlight, foundation color to the high points inside the oval: your forehead, under the eyes at the top of the cheekbones, and the tip of your chin. The eye will focus on these highlighted features first. So, if your face is too full, you'll be drawing attention to the narrow area in the middle of your face and away from the fuller sides.

3. Finally, apply your contour, or darkest shade, to the areas outside the oval: the temples and along your hairline and the sides of your cheeks, down to the jaw. By deepening the outside areas, you are making those areas visually recede and your face appear more narrow and oval.

4. If your skin is ivory/beige, you will contour your face more than you highlight, especially if you have really pale skin—the last thing you want to do is wash out your skin tone even more. Contouring, therefore, will give you the most dramatic change. If you have bronze/ebony skin, you will highlight your skin more than contour, especially if you have darker bronze/ebony skin tones. God gave you beautiful dark pigment in your skin; contouring will not really show. But what you highlight makes a huge difference, because it will brighten your skin and add life. So, again, my simple rule: Women with ivory/beige skin will contour more than highlight; women with bronze/ebony skin will highlight more than contour.

Once you've applied your three foundation shades, powder with a shade that matches your natural skin tone. The powder will not negate all the work you have just done, just set everything beautifully. If you want your results to be even more dramatic, you can finish with three shades of powder: one that matches your true foundation shade, one that matches your highlight shade, and a darker or bronzing powder to match your contour shade. This will reinforce your work and give you a beautifully sculpted effect that will make any face shape appear more oval and more youthful.

You'll finish with a pop of the perfect shade of blush on the apples of your cheeks, for that youthful glow, but we will get to that in Chapter 9. You can now see how adding depth (your contouring) and shape to the face can really make you look years younger.

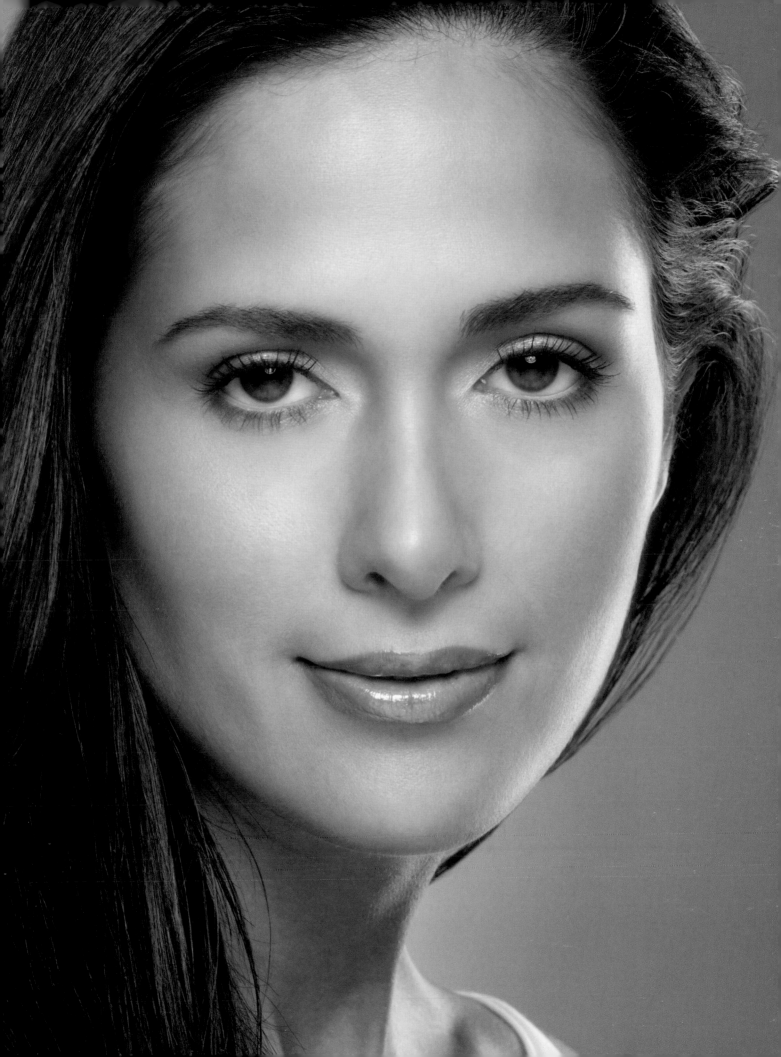

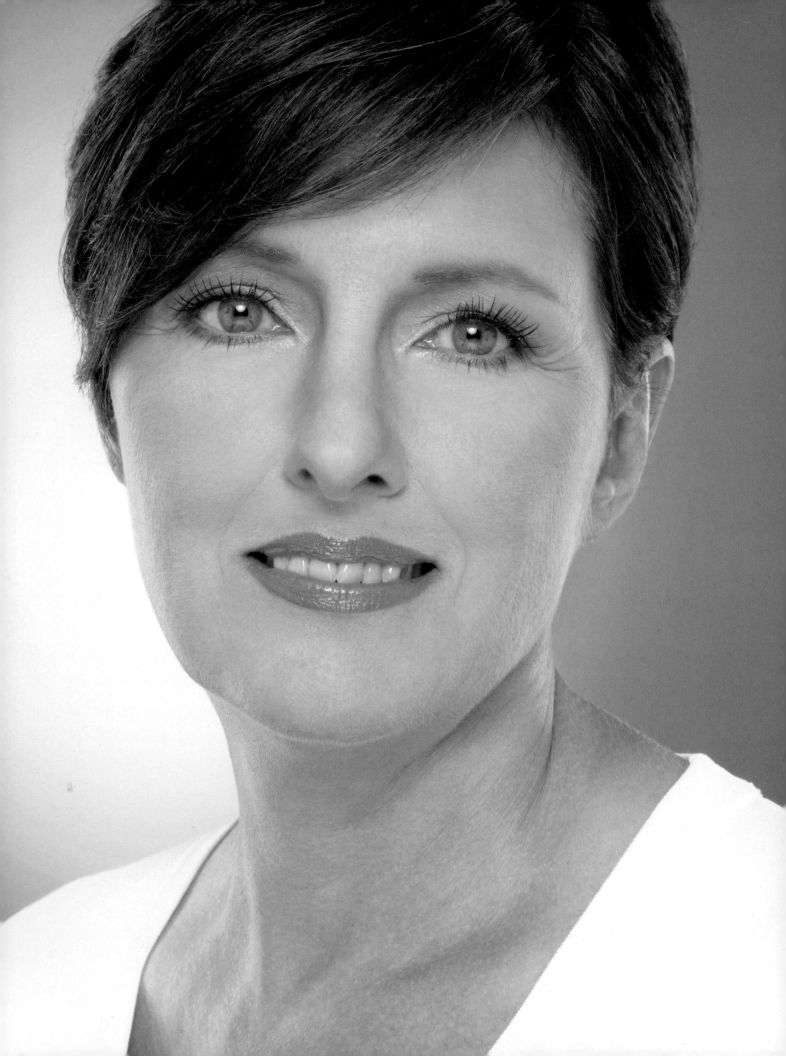

face shape

How the face is sculpted varies slightly with each face shape, but it always ends with the same results: looking younger and thinner. You do not need to know your exact face shape to make yourself look your absolute best—you might even have a combination of face shapes. All you really have to do is envision the oval, then highlight the high points inside the oval and contour what falls outside the oval.

Everything about your face is unique, including its shape, but no matter what the shape, you can add to it a youthful glow. You use the same components to sculpt every face shape, but you will adjust (customize) them for your own unique face. Let's start by looking at the best sculpting application for every face shape.

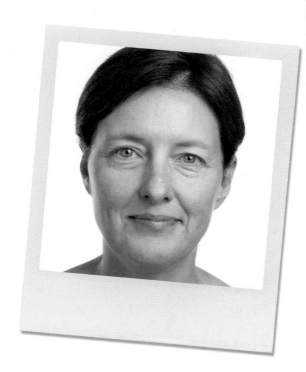

oval face

An oval-shaped face is considered by most people to be the perfect facial shape, because of its symmetry. It is usually broader at the cheeks, tapering in slightly at both the forehead and the chin. If you pictured an oval around your face and nothing extended past the oval, your face is oval. Because of its symmetry, you do not have to contour and highlight your face. This doesn't mean you wouldn't benefit from a generous dusting of bronzer along the cheekbones, temples, and even a bit on the tip of the chin. The bronzer will give you a glow and give your skin some life, making it look really youthful. You can experiment and play all you want. An oval face can support most makeup trends, so have fun!

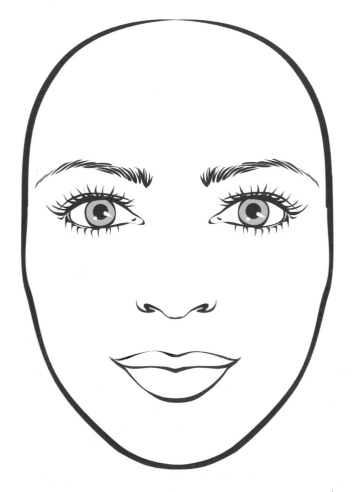

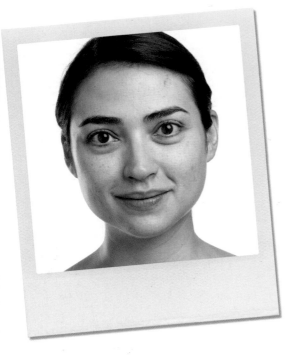

round face

A round face is fuller and generally holds its youthful appearance longer than other face shapes (definitely a plus!). It's shorter, fairly wide, with full cheeks and a rounded chin. When picturing your oval, some fullness will extend past the oval. Contouring that fullness away will create the illusion you are after. If you have a round face:

- Highlight your forehead, underneath the eyes just on top of the cheekbones, and the center of your chin to draw attention to the center of your face.

- Contour your temples, cheeks, and jawline with a bronzer or foundation that is one or two levels darker than your skin tone, to create the illusion of an oval.

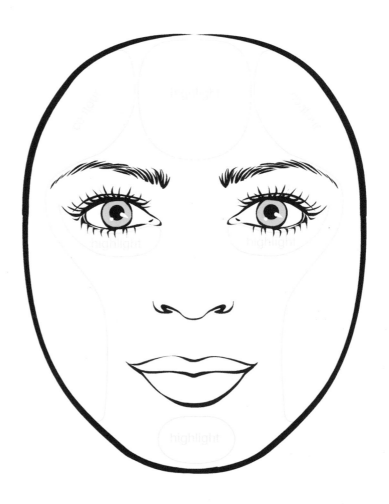

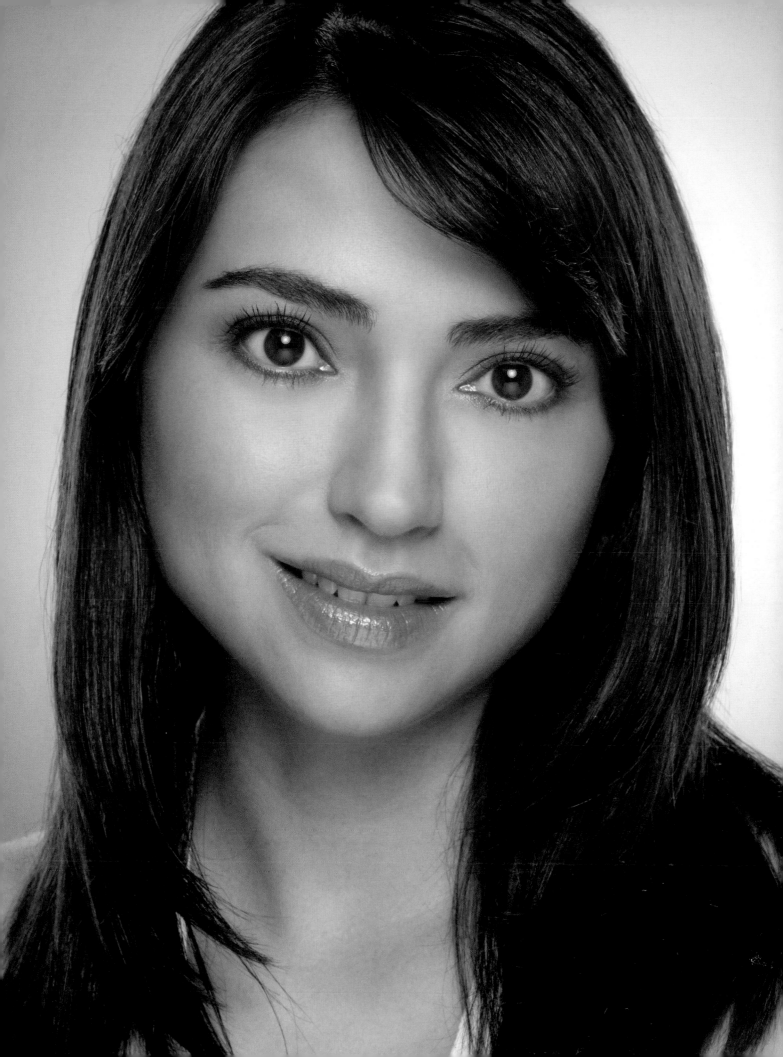

square face

I consider this shape to be one of the most beautiful because it suggests strength and the features are usually symmetrically balanced. A square face is the same width at the forehead, cheeks, and jaw. When envisioning your oval around this face shape, you will be left with four corners to contour or soften. If you have a square face:

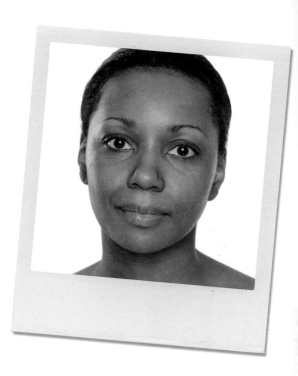

- Highlight down the center of your forehead, underneath the eyes just on top of the cheekbones, and the tip of your chin to draw attention to the middle of your face.

- Contour your hairline at the two corners by your temples and the jaw at the two corners.

- Apply blush on the apples of your cheeks, to help draw attention away from the corners of the square and help widen the area and make it appear more oval.

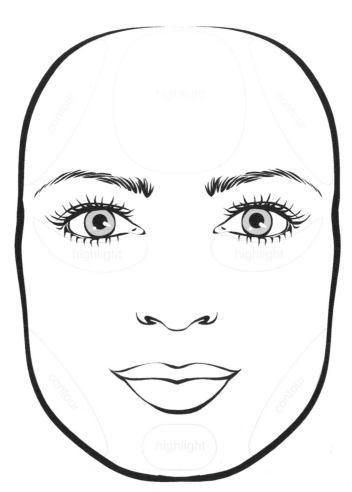

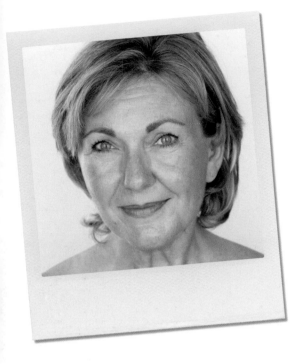

heart-shaped face

The heart-shaped face looks like an inverted triangle: it's wider at the forehead and cheeks, curving down to a narrow chin. When you picture your oval, you will notice a fullness extending at your temples and cheeks, so you should contour and soften the fullness in these areas. This is probably the least-common face shape. If you have a heart-shaped face:

• Highlight the chin to help broaden it. Highlight the forehead and underneath the eyes just on top of the cheekbones to draw attention to the center of your face.

• Contour the temples and cheeks to diminish the width of this portion of your face.

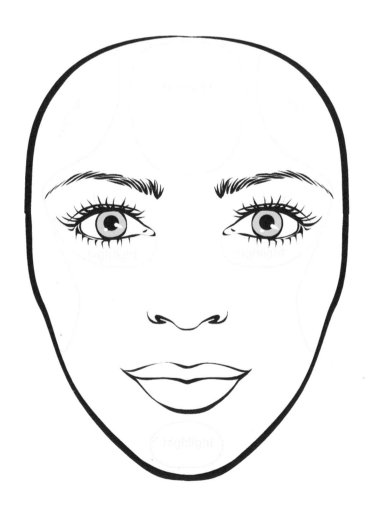

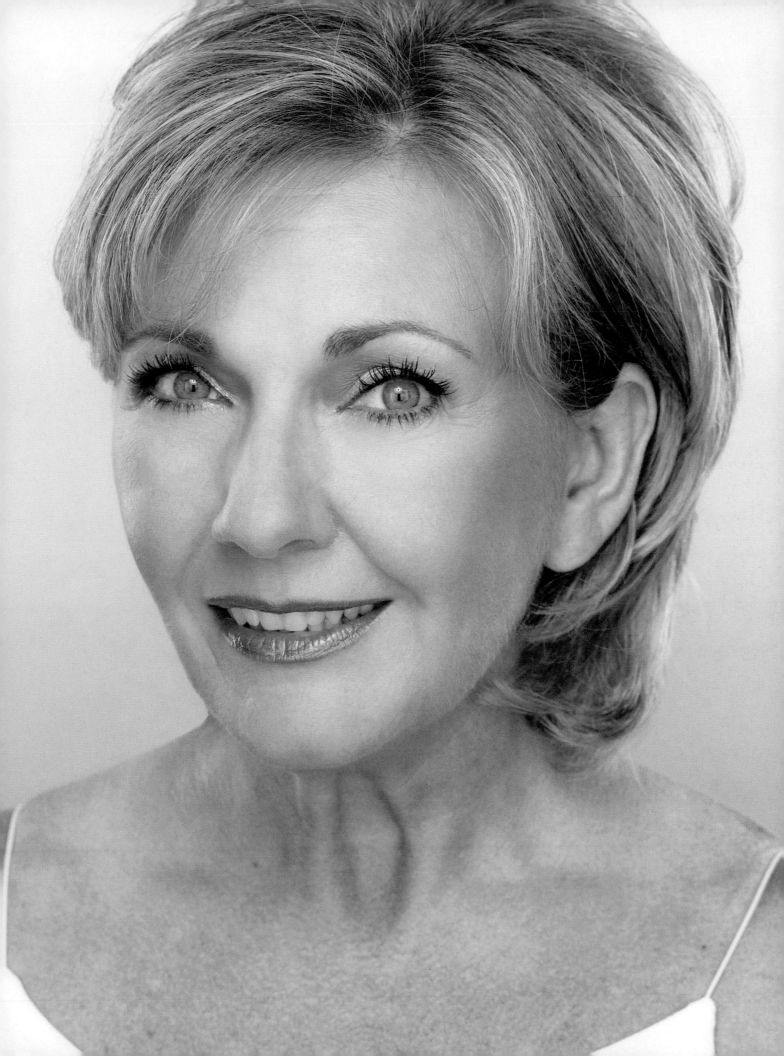

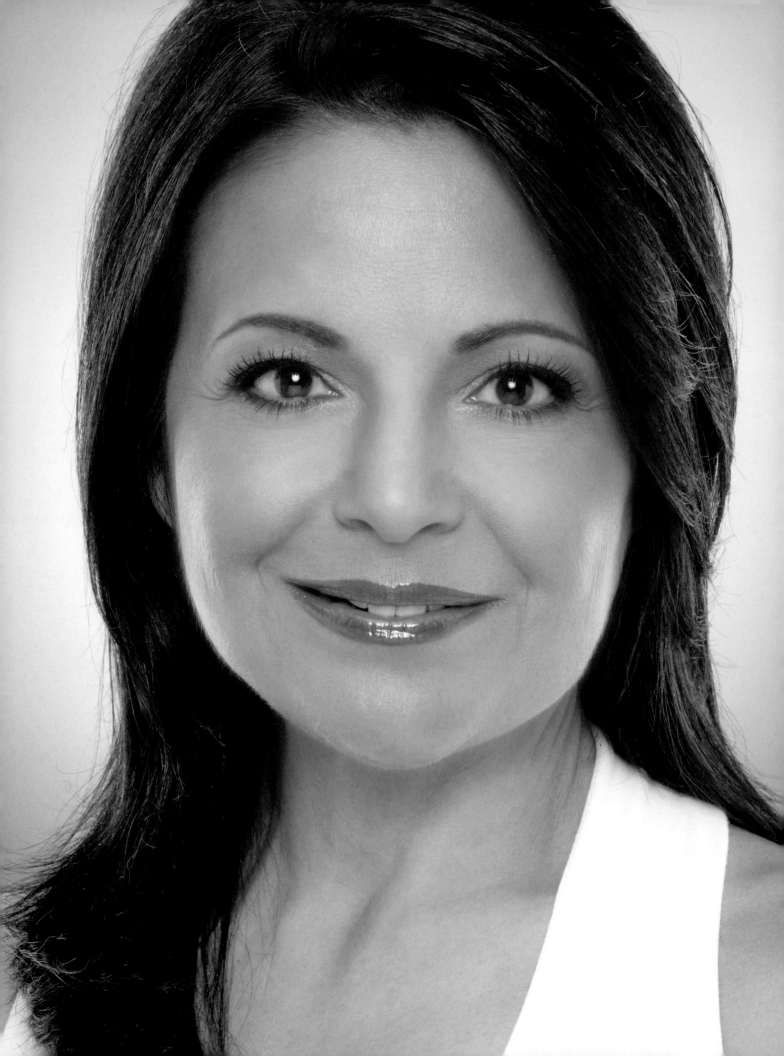

pear-shaped face

The pear-shaped face is narrow at the temples and forehead and wider at the cheeks and jawline. When envisioning your oval, your cheeks and jaw will extend past your oval, so this is the area you need to minimize. This is probably the most common face shape. If you have a pear-shaped face:

- Highlight your forehead to create the illusion of width, and highlight underneath the eyes on top of the cheekbones and the tip of your chin.

- Contour from your cheeks down along your jaw to minimize the width of this area.

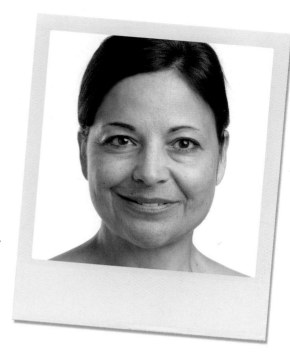

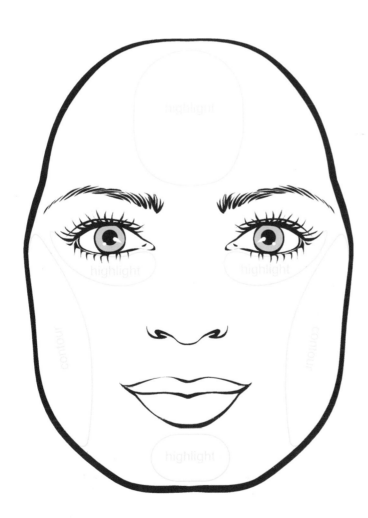

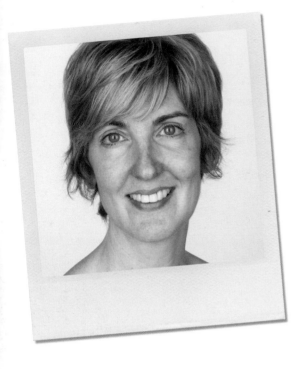

long face

The long face has high cheekbones, a high, deep forehead, and a strong, sharp, chiseled jawline. If you have a long face:

- Never highlight the oval area of your face! This will make your face appear even longer.

- Brush a bit of bronzer across your chin and across your forehead at your hairline to help make your face look shorter.

- Be generous with blush on the apples of your cheeks. This will help widen and shorten your face. When applying your blush, start closer in on the apples of the cheeks and brush outward across the face.

- Bangs can help shorten the length of your face as well.

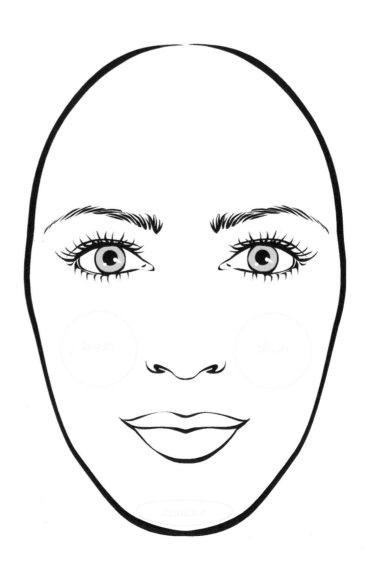

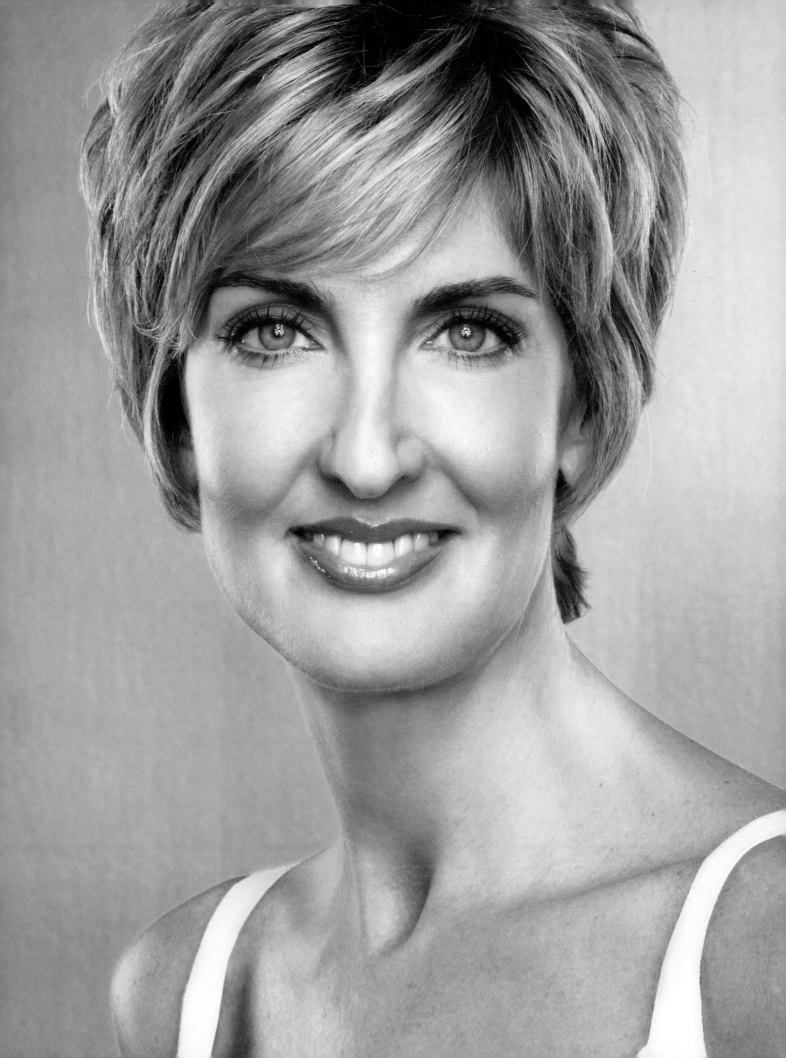

karen, 50s

I love Karen's features—I just couldn't see them. Smile and the world will smile back. I love that I was able to make such a beautiful woman even more beautiful.

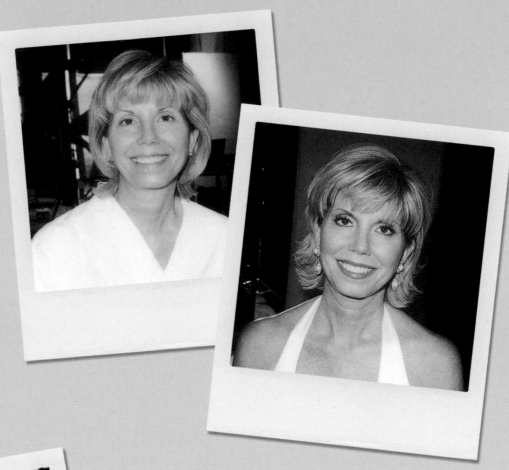

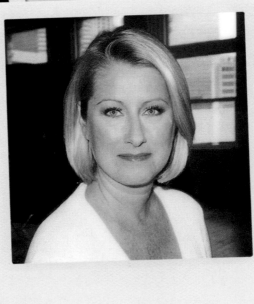

madeline, 40s

Madeline's features were invisible; they just fade away. I love how I was able to really make her gorgeous eye color pop. Evening out her skin was just what she needed.

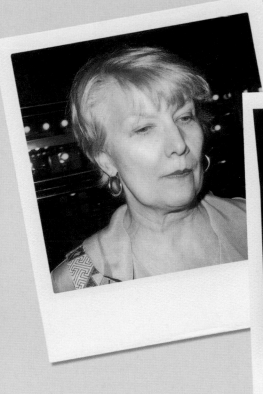

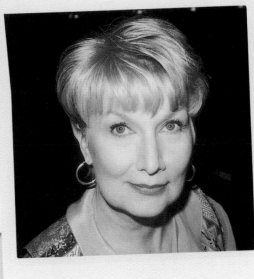

lori, 50s

All I could see was Lori's hidden potential. Talk about the benefit of adding color to the face! I love that I was able to unlock her hidden beauty.

janice, 40s

I could not focus on anything but how Janice's hair was aging her; a brush and blow dryer are her best friends. Now you can see her eyes, not her hooded eyelids.

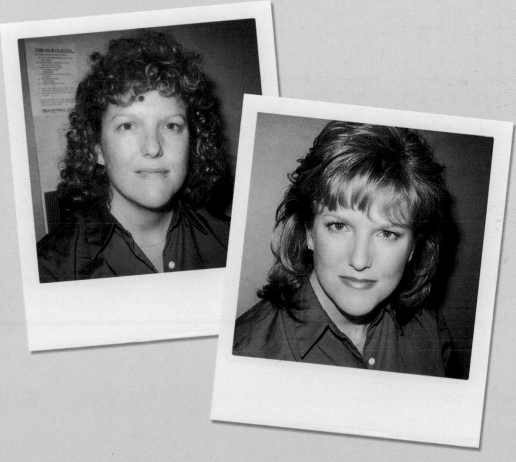

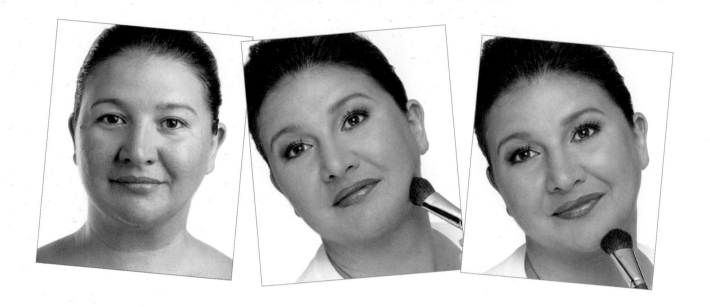

last-minute touches

laugh lines

Expression lines are commonly referred to as "laugh lines" and are most noticeable around the mouth. Laugh lines tend to deepen with age and can definitely make you look years older than you actually are. They tend to be genetic and can also be caused by environmental factors, such as sun damage and smoking. Although you can't completely get rid of laugh lines with makeup, you can certainly make them a lot less noticeable, and, by reducing their appearance, you will look younger.

Our *looking younger* secret weapon of choice for disguising laugh lines is a highlighting pen. The beauty of a highlighting pen is its lightweight formula and light-reflective properties, which bring forward recessed areas of the face. Because laugh lines become more visible as they deepen, highlighting in the crease of the line can make them less visible. To disguise them, first apply your foundation to create smooth, even-textured skin. Now, apply your highlighting pen along the entire length of the crease, from nose to mouth. Be sure to apply the pen just inside the crease, where it is creating a shadow. Then use your finger and stipple (a patting motion) along the highlighted area. This will blend in the color and minimize your laugh lines.

Q&A When I look in the mirror, I see more chins than I would like. How can I minimize the appearance of that fullness in a way that looks completely natural?

You can minimize the fullness very simply: After applying your makeup, use a narrow, slightly flat, dense brush and a matte bronzer (it should have no shimmer—the shine will accentuate the fullness, rather than reduce it) to apply a light layer of bronzer along your jawline. This gives the jawline greater definition, while lightly darkening the fuller area of skin making it appear to recede. Voilà—you have only one chin, instead of two! Avoid using a shade that is dramatically darker than your natural skin tone; one that's a couple of shades darker gives the most natural effect. Drawing attention up and away from the features you dislike is a definite move toward a youthful appearance.

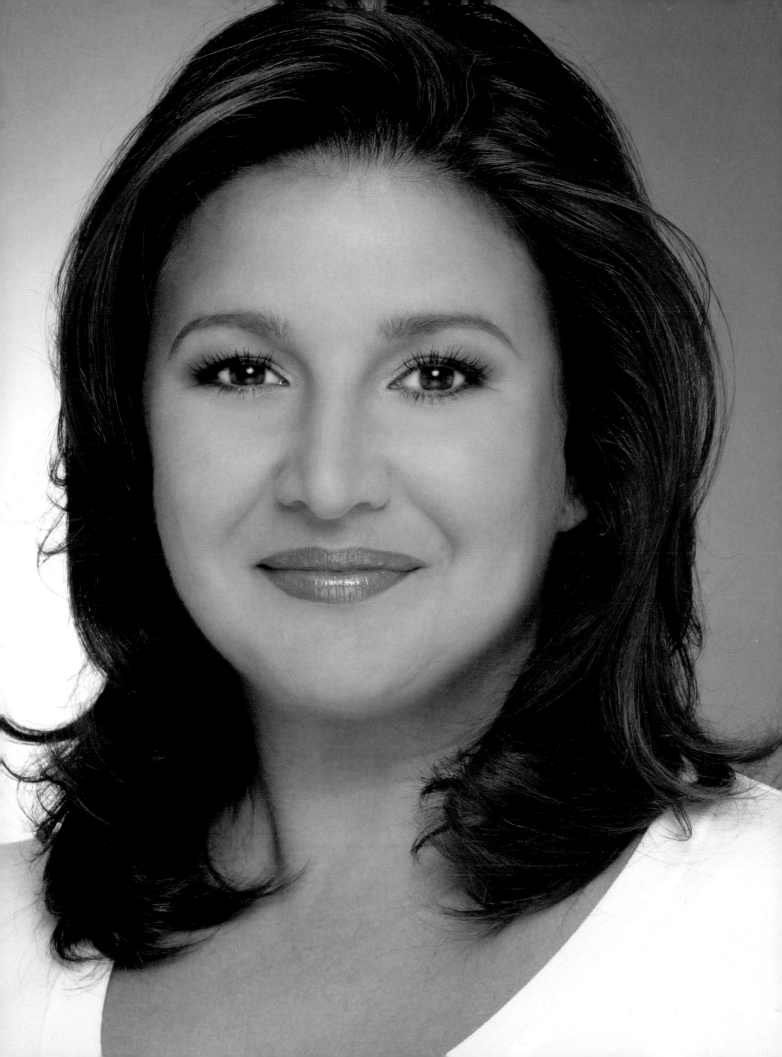

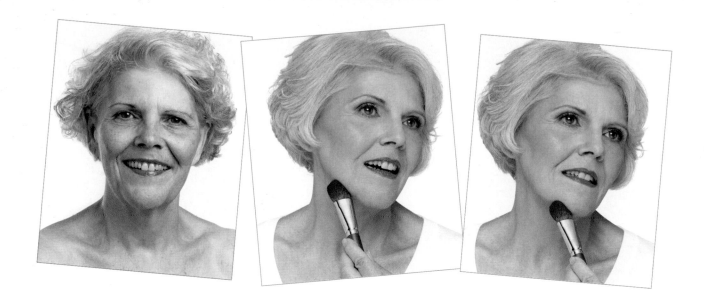

 The definition along my jawline has softened and is less taut and defined than it used to be, making me look less youthful. What can I do to recreate that youthful definition?

One of the signs of aging that people object to most is the softening (a slight drooping of the skin) of their jawline. Here is a quick, easy fix using makeup to recreate the definition of youth. When you have finished applying your makeup, use a narrow, slightly flat, dense brush and a matte bronzer (no shimmer, it will not look natural) and apply a light layer along your jawline. This gives your jawline more definition (giving you back your youthful jawline) and makes the droopy skin less visible. Something else to keep in mind is that anytime there is an area of you face you do not like, drawing attention away from it helps to minimize the flaw. For example, wearing a softer lip color and more intense eye makeup will help draw everyone's eye up and away from the lower area of your face, taking the focus away from what you do not want people to see. Whereas a dark or intense lip color draws everyone's eye to the area you want to minimize. Often, looking younger is about emphasizing the features you love about your face.

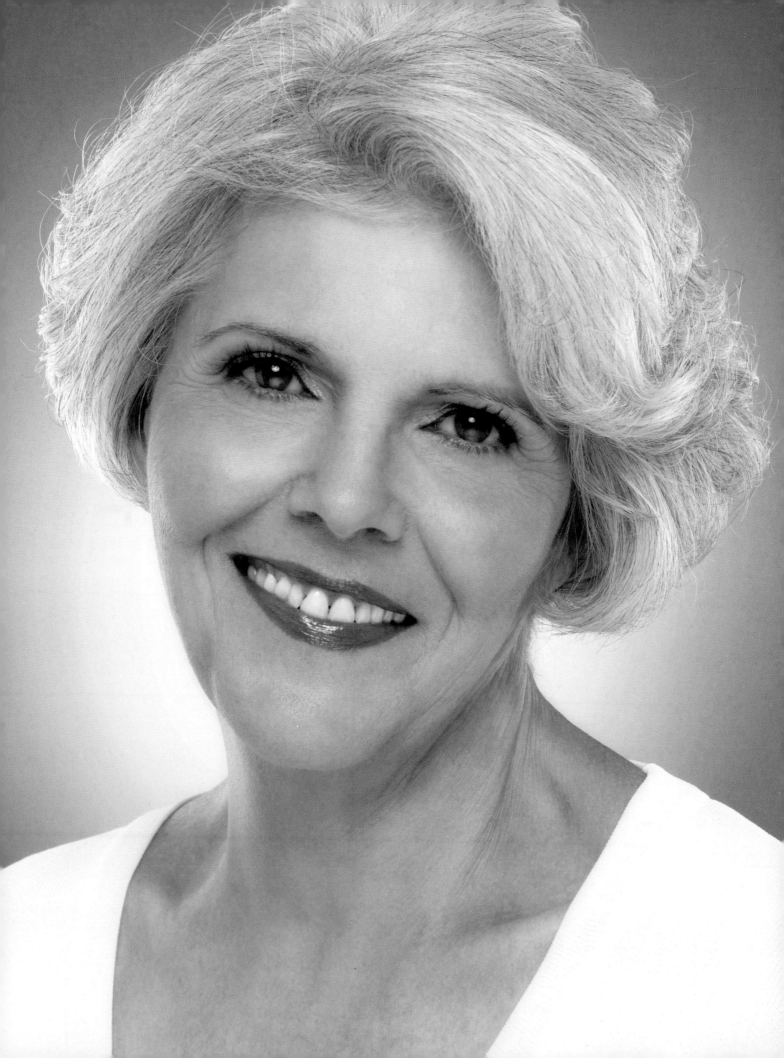

sunless tanning

By now, you should know that adding color to your skin is an effective way to look younger. Another option for adding color to your skin is sunless tanning, because we all know that the sun is not your best friend. However, the goal here is not to look like you just returned from weeks at the beach; you just want to give yourself a youthful glow.

Luckily, there are many formula options available, providing different degrees of color, so women with pale skin can choose a formula (shade) that gives less color, and those with a deeper skin tone can choose one that provides more color. You can also find formulas specifically designed for the face and for the body. The trick to getting a natural, realistic-looking result is being sure to build your color slowly, over time. You do not want one application to take you from pale to a deep-bronze goddess; you want to build your color gradually.

Here is the best way to achieve smooth, even coverage when applying self-tanning lotion:

1. Exfoliate well, using a product that will completely remove the top layer of dead, dry skin. This will help prevent areas of dry skin from becoming darker than the rest of your skin; dry skin soaks up more lotion, so it gets darker. Pay special attention to your elbows, hands, knees, ankles, and feet.

2. Moisturize your skin really well, to even out its porosity (your skin's ability to hold moisture). Concentrate on those areas you know are always the driest (your elbows, hands, knees, ankles, and feet).

3. For the face: Remember, we want to build color slowly. To help create a subtle, natural build of color, dilute the lotion by mixing equal parts self-tanning lotion with moisturizer and apply it to your face over a period of days. If you are very fair, you might want to mix two parts moisturizer with one part self-tanning lotion, so the

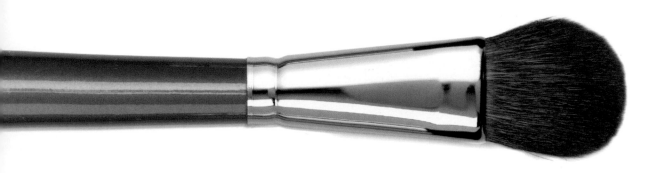

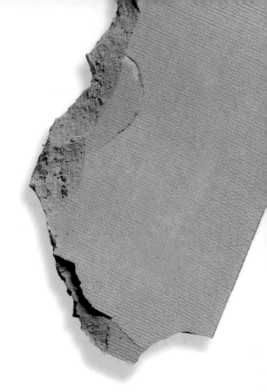

color build is even more subtle. This will help you gradually build your color over a period of time instead of in one application, so your skin will gradually start to glow and appear more natural.

Be sure to pour your self-tanner and moisturizer into a bowl and mix them completely before you start. Do not try to mix the two in your hands as you apply it—the solution will not go on evenly. If you have any dark spots, be sure to apply something such as Vaseline or a very thick, heavy moisturizer to the spots before applying the self-tanning lotion, and apply the sunless tanner around the spot, not on the spot. This prevents it from taking color and darkening as the rest of your skin tans. Do not forget to wash your hands really well immediately following your application, to prevent the sunless tanner from collecting and darkening around your knuckles and folds of your fingers.

You can find sunless tanning products that have already been mixed; these work well but can take longer to get the desired results. I find that, many times, creating your own formula can be the most effective way to achieve a more intense change. So, if you want ease and do not need an immediate shot of youth, go ahead and grab a premixed product. Keep in mind that, if you self-tan, you might need to adjust your foundation shade, so conduct another stripe test to keep your shade perfect.

4. For the body: Mix two parts self-tanner with one part moisturizer. Be sure to pour your self-tanner and moisturizer into a bowl and mix them completely before you start. Do not try to mix the two in your hands as you apply it—the solution will not go on evenly. If you are very fair, mix one part self-tanning lotion with one part moisturizer, to provide an even more subtle color change. Do not forget to wash your hands really well immediately following your application, to prevent the sunless tanner from collecting and darkening around your knuckles and folds of your fingers. I find that the best way to prevent this is to wear gloves when you apply the lotion. If you choose to tan your body and not your face, you will need to find a shade of foundation that you can blend along your jawline, to help your face match your neck and body.

nancy, 40s

Can you get past Nancy's amazingly beautiful blue eyes? I love those warm, coppery eyeshadow shades on blue eyes. Younger it is!

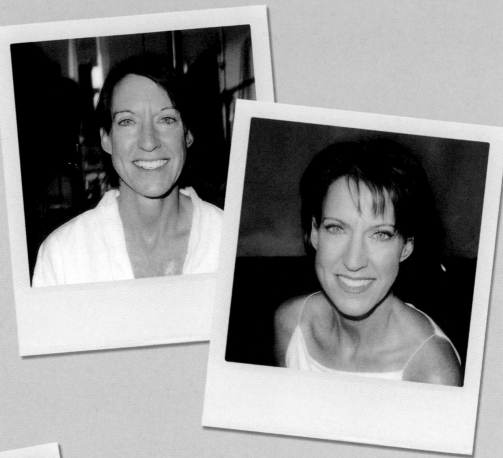

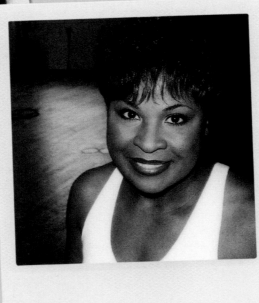

sonja, 40s

Flawless skin equals a younger look. I knew I could definitely make a difference. I loved that I gave Sonja a glow and was able to narrow her nose (the one thing she asked me to do).

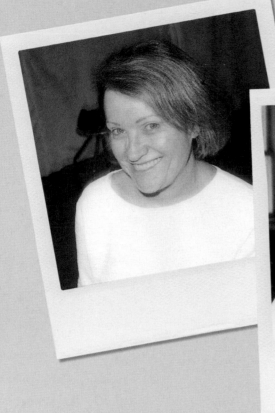

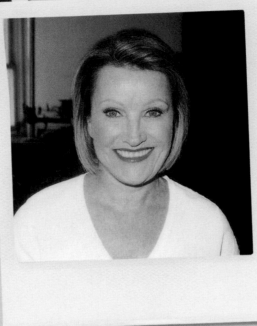

fran, 50s

I just wanted to soften and define Fran's features. I love that I was able to draw attention to her eyes and that contagious smile. Younger looking, for sure.

lynda, 50s

When I look at Lynda, all I can see is her inner beauty. I was so excited to be able to bring out what I saw inside. What gorgeous eyes.

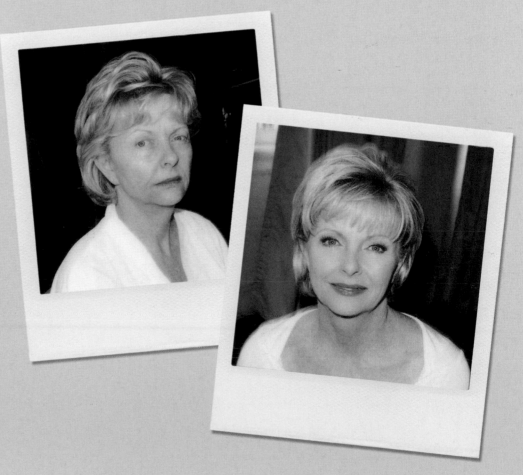

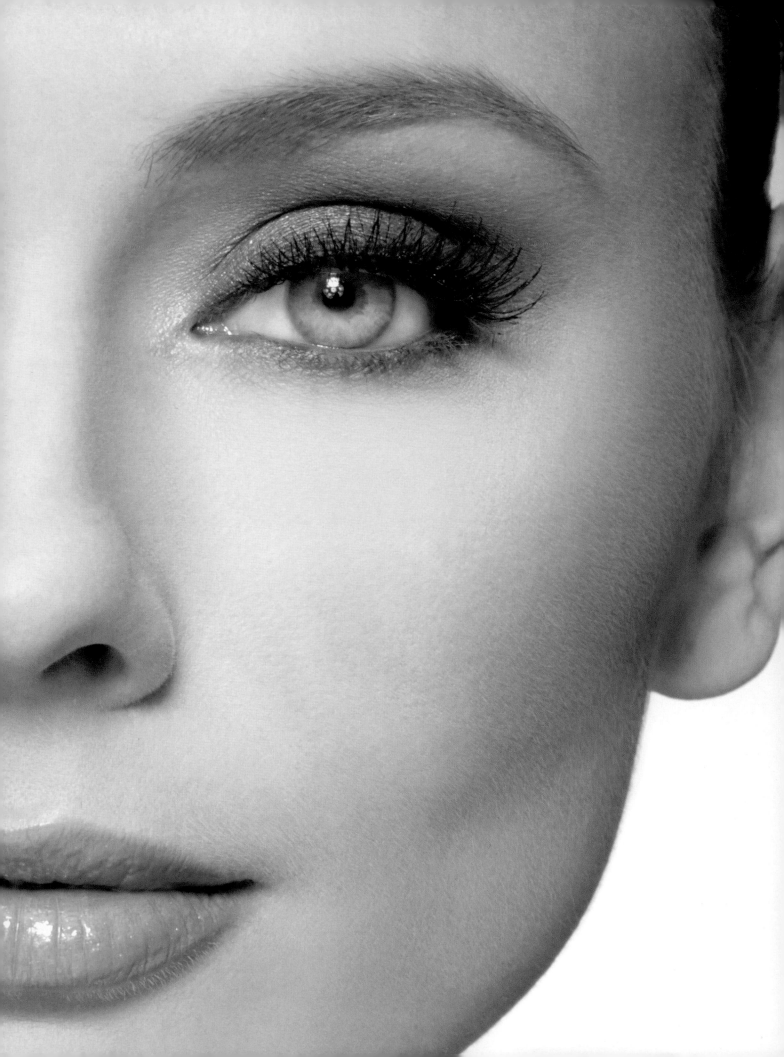

8

the eyes have it

It is often said that the eyes are the windows to the soul. If that is true, then what are yours saying about you? Applying color correctly to your eyes can go a very long way toward making your signature statement to the world. With eye makeup, your goal should always be to bring out your eyes and help them grab everyone's attention. When someone looks at you, you want that person to say that you look beautiful today, not that your eye makeup does.

There are definite dos and don'ts for applying eye makeup. In this chapter, you'll learn the tricks for applying color to your eyes and eyebrows. I will arm you with all the information you need to make the right color choices, as well as where and how to apply your eye makeup. Choosing the correct colors is important, because they will help you not only look your best but also look younger. Certain shades are much more forgiving and will make you look more youthful.

Equally important is the application, because with the proper application, you can accentuate the aspects you want people to see, such as beautiful eye color or long lashes, while drawing their attention away from what you do not want them to see—wrinkles or crepey lids, for example. You can make yourself look more alive and awake.

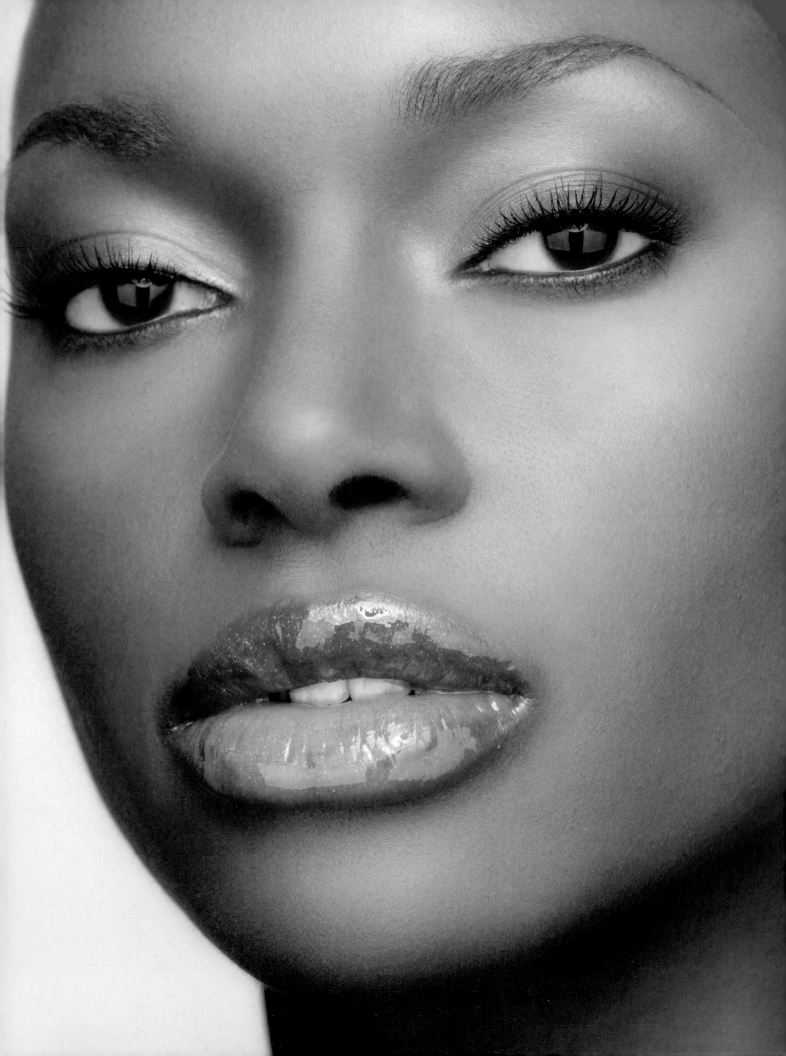

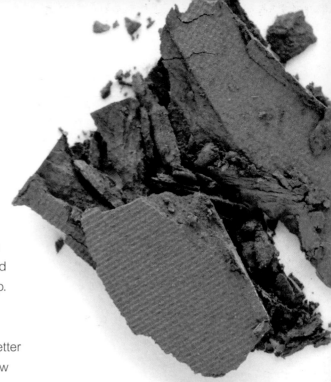

change is good

Throughout this chapter, I will share with you all kinds of application techniques. Remember that practice makes perfect. Don't be scared to try something new! After all, you can't harm yourself with makeup. If you don't like the way your makeup looks, simply wash it off and start over. So, feel free to play and try new things!

Your look should change over time. Products change and get better with new technology; by sticking with the same old thing forever, how will you discover the new and improved products that might work better for you? Unfortunately, it is human nature to stop changing once we feel we have reached our most beautiful (for most women, this is in their thirties). But sticking with a look you have been wearing since 1992 actually ages you. Your look has to grow and change as you get older if you want to look your most youthful, no matter what your age.

brows

Did you know that you can choose a brow color as easily as a hair color? It's true, and you should take advantage of it, especially when you're trying to look younger. When selecting a brow color, the basic rule of thumb is that it should pretty closely match your hair color (whether natural or chosen). Let's elaborate a little bit, though, because as you know, it is just not as simple as that. Here are the perfect brow colors for each hair color:

- **light blonde:** same shade as hair or one shade darker
- **medium** to **dark blonde:** same color as hair
- **auburn:** same color as hair
- **light brown:** same color as hair or one shade lighter
- **medium** to **dark brown:** same color as hair or one shade lighter
- **very dark brown** to **black:** one shade lighter than your hair color
- **silver** or **grey:** use a blonde or soft taupe color for ivory or beige skin tones, and use a light golden brown for bronze or ebony skin tones (a silver or grey brow color to match your hair would just wash you out and make you look older)

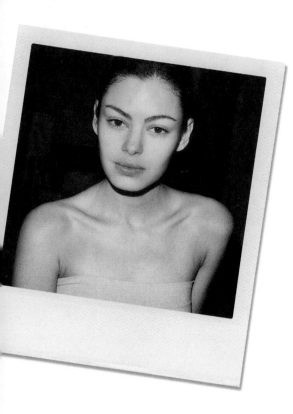

Our *looking younger* secret is that softer-colored brows make you look younger. Very dark, harsh brows can be aging, so when in doubt, always go a shade lighter. I would rather see a woman walking around with brows that are too light than looking like she has two dark slashes above her eyes.

Many women with silver or grey hair may still have dark brows (probably because their hair was dark when they were younger). But, trust me, you want to fill them in with a softer, lighter brow color, to soften the brows' appearance and make you look younger. In fact, a blonde or taupe shade on ivory/beige skin will help define and soften your brows, while helping them blend better with your hair and face, even if your natural brow color is dark. For bronze/ebony skin, choose a light golden brown, instead of the dark brown your brows were originally. This will soften your brows' final look and help you look more youthful.

Just a reminder: Brow color products are specifically designed for the job. Brow pencils are duller in color, usually with no sheen, and have a waxier texture than eyeliner pencils. Eyebrow powder is duller and more matte than eyeshadow. So be sure to use products designed to do the job.

application

When applying brow color, the goal is to mimic your natural brows. You want to apply the color in short, feather-like hair strokes, never in a straight, solid line. The short feather-like hair strokes are meant to imitate natural brow hairs.

As we learned in Chapter 3 (page 29), you have multiple brow color products from which to choose. Let's review the different types of brow color and grooming products and the best application technique for each.

tip:

When you have your hair colored, ask your colorist to tint your brows to match. This will ensure that your brow color matches your hair color.

pencil

A brow pencil is probably the most commonly used and most portable coloring tool. The sharper the point, the better the application, so sharpen your pencil before you start.

1. Apply your pencil using short, feathery, hair-like strokes, angled in the same direction as the hairs' growth. Your strokes should mimic natural brow hairs (never draw a solid, straight line).
2. Using a small, stiff, angled brush, go over the pencil strokes you just applied, using the same short strokes. This will blend your color even more and make it look completely natural.

powder

Powder is the most natural-looking and easiest of all brow color to apply. It is perfect if your brows don't need much filling in, but you want to define and refine them. It is also the quickest and easiest to apply, because there is only one step: you apply and blend at the same time. Simply dip your short, stiff, angled brush in the product and apply it to your brows in short, feathery, hair-like strokes angled in the same direction as the hairs' natural growth. Remember: no straight lines, just short, feathery strokes.

crème

Crème provides the most coverage, but it is not my brow color of preference, because it is the hardest to make look natural. However, it might be a good choice if you need a lot of coverage due to over-plucking or chemotherapy. (You can also try the powder-on-pencil technique I discuss in "more coverage" on the next page.) Here's the best way to apply crème, for a natural look:

1. Using a short, stiff, angled brush, apply your crème using short, feathery, hair-like strokes.
2. Be sure to always follow your crème with powder brow color, using the exact same application method. The powder will set the crème and help it last all day.

tips:

Sharpen your brow pencil each time you use it. The sharper the point, the better the application.

You can use eyebrow pencil and eyebrow powder separately, or you can combine them. Layering them gives you more complete coverage and helps the color last longer and look more natural.

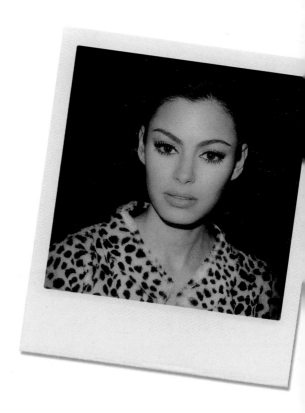

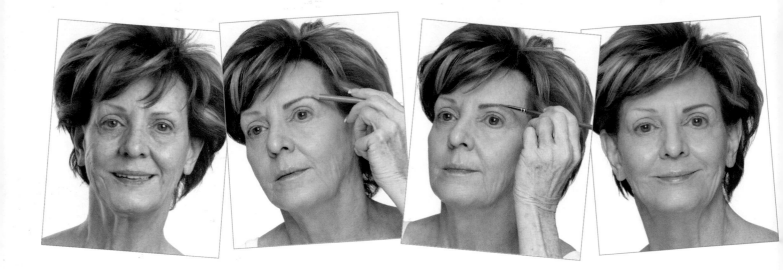

more coverage

If you have scars in your brows or brows that just are not there, you will need more coverage. You could use a crème, but I prefer to layer brow pencil and brow powder together, because I feel that it looks the most natural.

1. Apply your pencil using short, feathery, hair-like strokes, angled in the same direction as the hairs' growth. The strokes are meant to mimic natural brow hairs (never draw a solid, straight line).

2. Using a small, stiff, angled brush, go over the pencil, using the same short strokes. This will blend your color and help it to look natural.

3. Dip your brush into your brow powder and apply as before, using short, feathery, hair-like strokes angled in the same direction as the hairs' growth. Be sure to cover the entire brow. The powder and pencil layered together provide more complete coverage and help the color last longer and look more natural.

finishing touches

Regardless of the method you prefer for grooming your brows, always finish by using a brow brush (my favorite is shaped like a toothbrush) to brush your brow hairs upward and outward. This ensures that your brow hairs lie in place and that your color blends beautifully for an absolutely natural effect. If you have wild, unruly brows and need help keeping them tamed during the day, you can finish with a brow gel. It acts like hairspray for the brows. To review how to best shape your brows, turn to page 76.

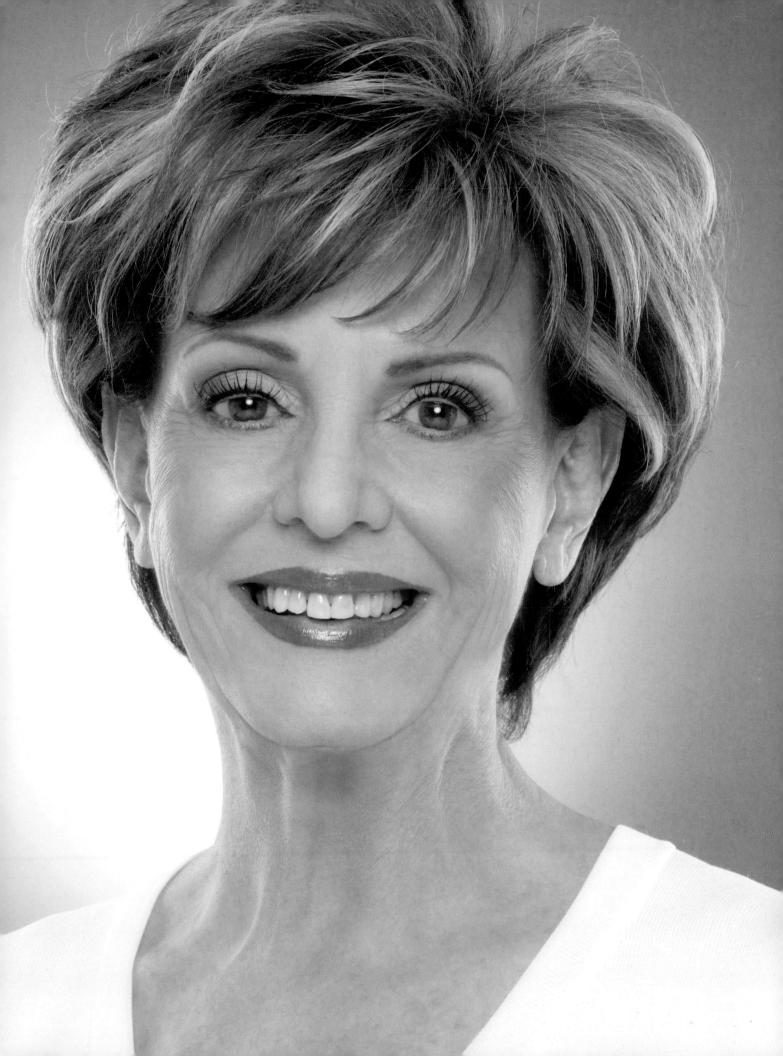

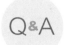**Q&A**

My brows have thinned out so much over the years. Is it true that fuller brows make you look younger? How can I make them look fuller but still natural?

Yes, fuller brows do make you look younger, and brows do thin naturally as you age. I think part of the reason for this is that they do not remain as high as they use to be, and, as they drop, they thin out (just my personal theory). You can add fullness back to your brows by layering on pencil and powder. This will give you more coverage, look more natural, and help the color last longer. Use the "more coverage" technique discussed on page 158.

I am not letting my hair go grey, but I am starting to get flecks of grey in my brows. I try to cover them with pencil and powder, but nothing really covers the grey. If I tweeze them, my brows are too sparse. Do I have any other option for covering grey hairs in my brows?

Yes—you can have them professionally tinted. Visit a salon that tints brows and have them colored. There are special and specific tints designed just for the eye area, and they can completely cover the grey hairs. But, please, have this done by a professional who knows what he or she is doing: Do *not* do it yourself at home!

I have a lot of brow hairs, but they are so light that you can't see them. When I apply my brow pencil it always looks unnatural, because my natural blonde brow hairs lie over the pencil, causing it to look fake. What can I do so that my brows are defined yet appear natural?

The answer for you is tinting your brows, so that they will show. Have a professional at a salon darken your brows with a product designed specifically for use in the eye area. This color tends to fade quickly, so consider having your brows tinted a shade darker than you want—the color will last longer. Once your brows are tinted, you will need less brow pencil, and what you do use will look completely natural.

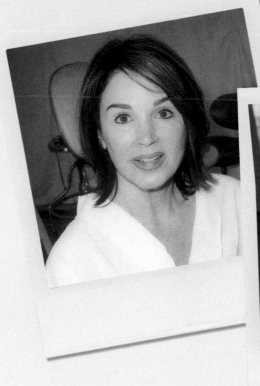

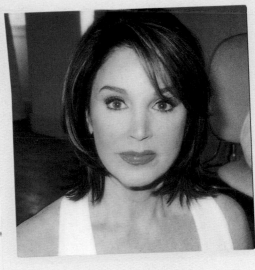

lana, 50s

Lana is naturally beautiful, but the right definition makes a big difference. A beautiful glow, defined eyes, and luscious lips—now that makes gorgeous.

gayle, 30s

Gayle has amazing eyes and beautiful lips; they just needed a little definition. Applying a soft, subtle color to her lips but still creating definition created an immediate youthfulness. The right color choice is paramount for making this happen.

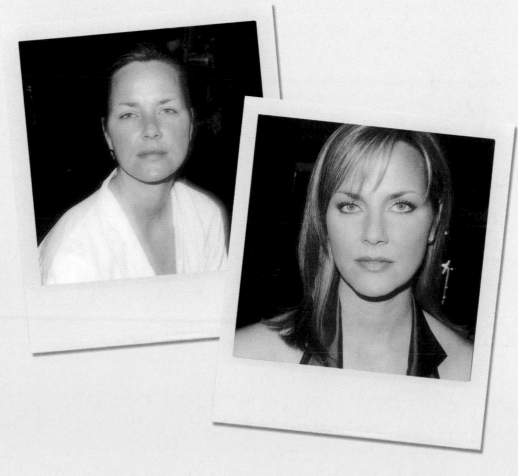

eyes

To me, the eyes are so important that I seem to always (or at least 99 percent of the time) make them the focus of the face. I think it is because I truly believe they are the windows to the soul. Your goal with eye makeup is to open up, lift, and make the eyes appear their most youthful. To achieve this, we need to consider a couple of key factors. The first is shape: Where do we need to apply your eyeshadow and eyeliner to really bring out your eyes and open them up? The second is eye color: Which shades of eyeshadow and eyeliner will best enhance and intensify your color? I want people to say, "your eyes look beautiful," not "your eyeshadow looks pretty." Makeup is always about enhancing your personal beauty.

Let's first talk about how to choose the right shades of eyeshadow and eyeliner. Following is a short list of what to consider when making your color choices.

eye color

The most important thing to think about when choosing eyeshadow and eyeliner is your own eye color. You want to select shades that will bring out the natural color of your eyes. Your goal is to make your eye color pop and stand out, not for your eyeshadow to compete with or diminish your natural color.

Need help selecting eyeshadow shades to enhance your natural eye color? The chart on page 164 will help guide you. Notice that I do not suggest blue shades for blue eyes or green shades for green eyes. The key is to select a shade that is the opposite of your eye color. For example, for blue eyes, choose a warm shade of brown or tawny or golden shades. Whenever you pair two opposite colors, they intensify each other. (This is a theory discovered and proven by Leonardo da Vinci, so I am not making it up.) Using shades of eyeshadow or eyeliner that are the opposite of green (coppery, warm browns or purple) will make the green in the iris of your eyes look brighter and much more green.

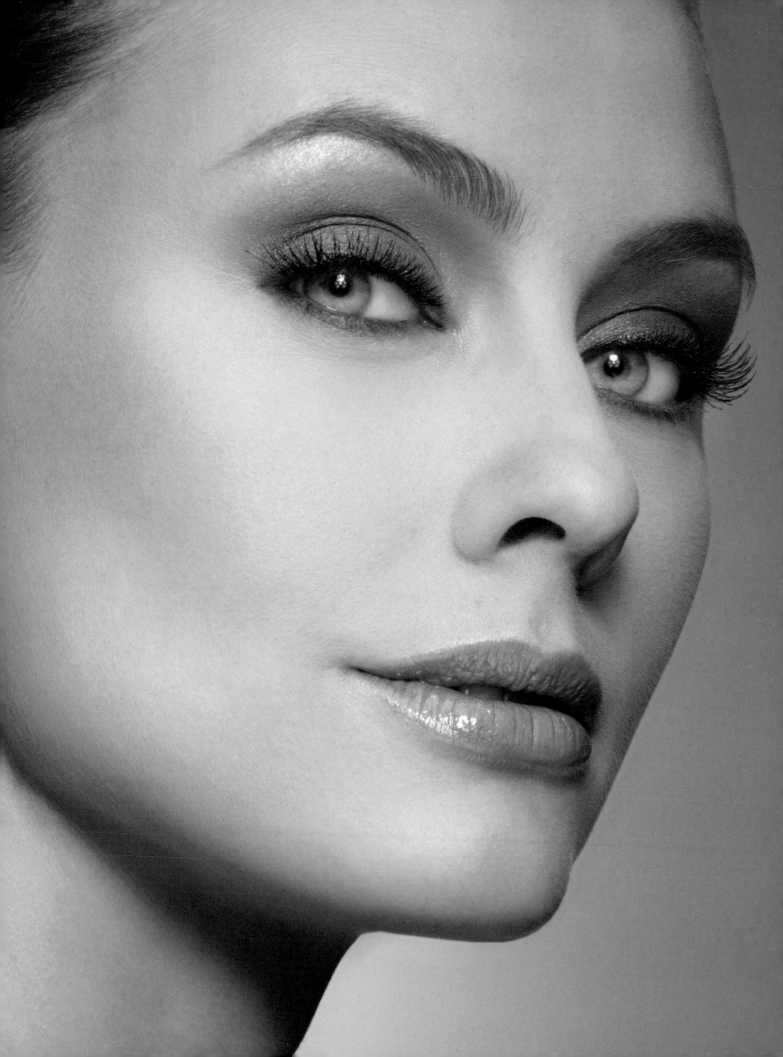

eye color	liner	eyeshadow
blue	warm brown bronze taupe burgundy black	golden brown warm taupe copper golden khaki rich raisin charcoal
green	warm brown bronze taupe purple burgundy black	warm brown rich taupe dark purple coppery bronze deep burgundy soft violet charcoal
brown	rich brown bronze dark taupe rich purple burgundy navy black	golden brown mahogany coppery bronze dark purple deep espresso rich blue deep green pewter charcoal
grey	deep brown black steel grey	charcoal cool brown deep burgundy pewter

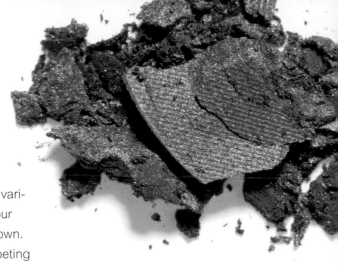

If you have brown eyes, lucky you! You can experiment with a variety of colors and still enhance your natural eye color. So play to your heart's content with purple, green, gold, navy, silver, copper, or brown. Any color looks beautiful around brown eyes; you will not be competing with your natural eye color.

If you are wondering why you do not see a category on the chart for hazel eyes, it is because hazel eyes are not a single color. Hazel eyes are a mixture of colors, either green and brown or green and blue. Choose the eye color you want to enhance, and refer to the corresponding color category. If you have blue-green hazel eyes, for example, you can choose shades from the blue or green category. If you have green-brown hazel eyes, you can choose colors from the green or brown category. You get to pick; don't be afraid to experiment.

You will see that there is a grey category. I think of this as a pale eye color. It can be pale blue or pale green, but what makes it special is that the iris of the eye is always surrounded by a dark ring. So, surrounding this eye color with rich, deep eyeshadow and eyeliner colors will make your eyes glow.

I do need to make one really important point: It is true that, as you age, softer colors are better, because darker shades can be harsh and aging. They do not have to be dull, subtle, and boring, but you will want to lighten the depth level of your color choices as the years go by. Stay in the same color family, to bring out your eye color, but instead of a deep, dark brown, go with a soft deep bronze. Your shades can have depth—they just do not need to be really intense and dark.

When choosing eyeliner, follow the same rules for choosing eyeshadow. I will say, though, that I think natural, neutral shades (bronze, brown, black, and charcoal) do more for defining your eyes than bright colors—although I do love a deep burgundy liner with every eye color as well. You can feel free to play with color if it is appropriate for your eye color. Just remember, if you want more definition, the more basic shades will give it to you.

tip:

If you have mature skin, be sure to choose eyeshadow shades with a matte finish—a matte finish draws less attention to fine lines and looks the most natural.

skin tone

Skin tone is another factor to consider when choosing your eyeshadow. By skin tone, I mean the depth level of your skin. Your shade choices will make a difference in the intensity of your look. Women with dark ebony skin might want to steer clear of eyeshadows that are too white or light. Likewise, women with fair, pale skin should avoid eyeshadows that are too dark, unless they want a really dramatic look. I prefer a more natural look (especially for women who want to look younger), so I usually choose shades that tend toward neutral (at least for daytime) and aren't too high in contrast to your skin's depth level. Save your dramatic looks for those special evenings out.

matching

Although some women think they should, you do *not* have to match your eye makeup to your clothing. Makeup—like your clothing—is an accessory to *you*. Makeup is *not* an accessory to your clothing. Matching your makeup colors to your clothes can wash you out and might not always flatter your best features. The theory of opposites complementing each other applies here, too. Choose what looks best on you. When you choose your makeup shades, imagine that you're wearing white. This will help you choose shades that complement you, and your real beauty will shine through, instead of taking a back seat to your clothing or eye makeup.

I have very dark circles, which I think I do a really good job of hiding, but some eyeshadow colors seem to make them more noticeable, even after I have covered them. Is it my imagination, or am I seeing things?

No, you are not seeing things! It is true that, even after you have concealed severe discoloration, certain shades of eyeshadow can draw attention back to the area you just covered. For example, if you have extreme dark, bluish purple circles, you will want to stay away from shades of purple or blue eyeshadow and eyeliner, which will draw attention back to the circles. If you have covered really dark circles, choose a lighter shade of eyeshadow or eyeliner to define the lower lash line, so you don't reinforce the circles.

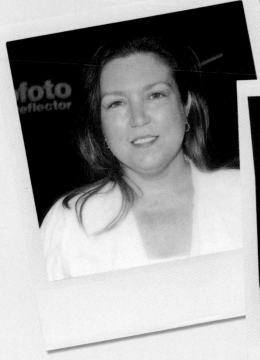

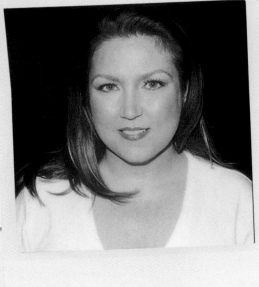

tracey, 40s

Tracey has beautiful cheekbones. The glow I created with the right blush is perfection. Also, defining her eyes and making them a feature was a great choice.

joy, 30s

All I could see were the possibilities, amazing features. I'm really so proud of what I achieved with Joy's eyes. I cannot stop looking at them. What a spark.

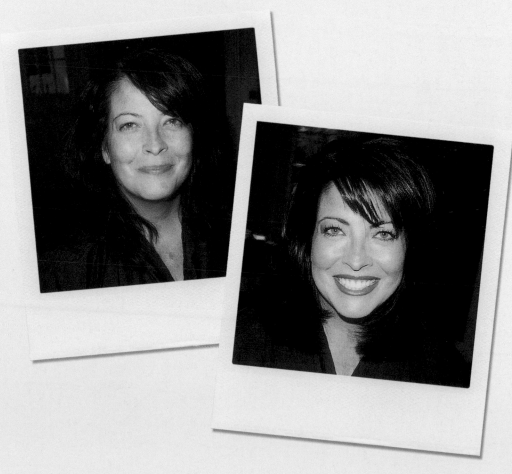

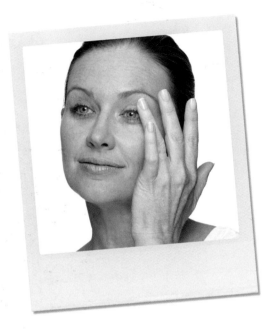

How can I get my eyeshadow to blend better, go on more smoothly, and last longer?

I always apply concealer and powder to eyelids before applying eyeshadow. They will cover discoloration on your eyelid and provide a clean canvas onto which you can artfully paint your eyeshadow. This technique also helps make your shades look clearer and more true in tone and helps your eyeshadows blend more easily and wear longer. I know some people think foundation will work for this, but some formulas can cause your eyeshadow to crease and will not cover discoloration nor create a clean canvas the way a concealer will.

Also available are products called eye primers, which can create a perfect surface for your shadow color; they help prevent creasing and keep the natural oils in your eyelids from reacting with the eyeshadows and causing them to build up in the crease. If you use an eye primer, you should still follow it with concealer and powder, because the primer will not cover all discoloration and can hinder the all-important blendability of your eyeshadows.

eyeshadow: basic application

You want to achieve two things when applying your eye makeup. The first is to give your lid shape by visually "pushing away" the areas you don't want to see and "bringing forward" the areas you do want to see. The second is to define and open up your eyes, which is greatly helped by achieving your first goal. Proper application makes your eyes appear more open and awake, and this can make you look years younger. This is why I first discuss eyeshadow application for the basic eye shape, and then move on to discuss application techniques for every other eye shape. The techniques for all eye shapes are similar, because the three key ingredients are the same; you just slightly adjust their placement, according to each individual eye shape.

To shape the eye, you use three shades: a highlight, a midtone, and a contour. The basic rule to remember is that everything you highlight will visually come forward and become more prominent, and everything you contour or darken will recede, or move away from you. Although there are thousands of shades from which to choose, for the best results, use the three-shade application technique. It will bring out your most beautiful features and draw attention to your eyes.

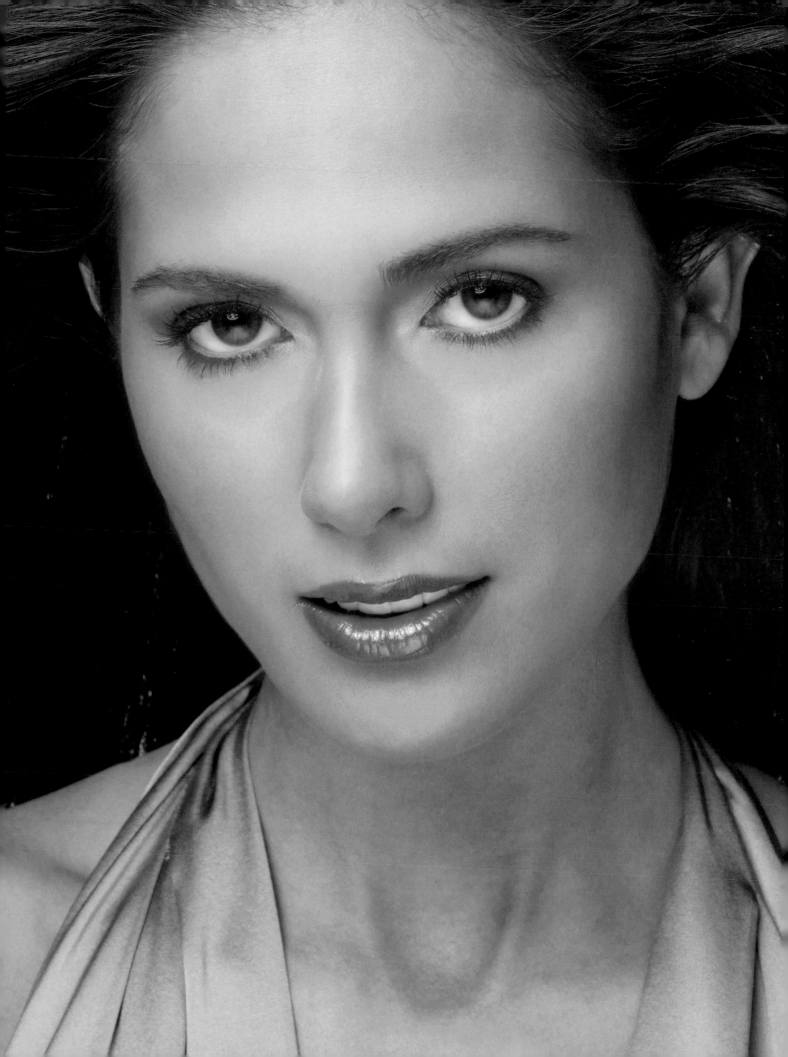

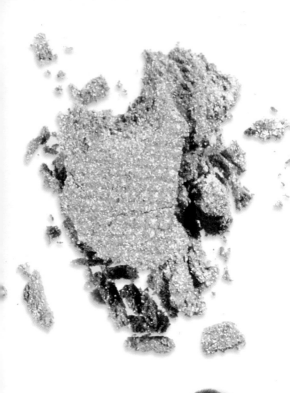

highlight

Your highlight shade is the lightest of the three eyeshadows. Everything you highlight visually comes forward. Your shade choice can be more or less dramatic, depending on the finish and the shade you select. A matte finish provides a much more subtle look than a shimmer finish. The shimmer is more dramatic. For example, I usually use a shimmer highlight on deep-set eyes, because it opens up the eye more than a matte shade. Lighter highlight shades are also more dramatic than soft or flesh-toned shades. How much you want to pull an area forward depends on whether you make a more or less dramatic shade choice.

Once you've chosen a highlight shade, apply it to your brow bone (the area immediately underneath your brow's arch) and your eyelid. Do not apply it all the way from the lash line to the brow, because such a sweeping application can be unflattering to your eye shape. Also apply your highlight shade to the inside corner of the lower lash line (visit page 56 to find the perfect brushes). This will really help open up your eyes, making them appear larger and more youthful.

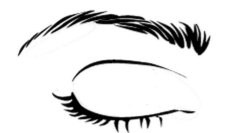

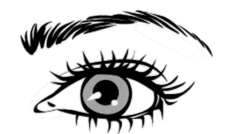

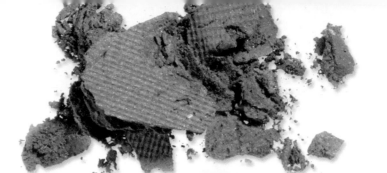

midtone

Your midtone shade is the most important shade, but can also be the most boring. The middle shade of your three eyeshadow colors, it is deeper than your highlight shade and lighter than your contour shade. It's the first step in the blending process and in creating definition in the crease of the eye. This shade should be the most natural—an extension of your skin tone. You'll change your highlight and contour colors more often than your midtone shade. Generally, your midtone color should have a matte finish, but it does not always have to be matte. A matte finish gives the lid a subtle, natural appearance. Your midtone starts the reshaping of your eyelids, because everything we add depth to will visually recede.

To apply it, start from the outside corner of the eyelid, because the first place you lay your brush receives the highest concentration of color. Gently move your brush along the crease of the eyelid, from the outside corner all the way across to the inside corner (visit page 56 for the perfect brush; my brush #29 is the perfect shape for applying midtone color). For a very defined crease, you can apply a few more layers of your midtone shade (feel free to layer for more definition), always making sure to blend it where it meets the highlight shade. Then, take your midtone shade and apply it along your lower lash line. As before, start your application from the outside corner, sweeping your brush; across to the inside corner (again visit page 56 to find the perfect brush; my brush #13 will give you the application you need). Applying midtone here before you apply eyeliner or contour shade helps create a blend, because you are building depth of color.

tips:

If you're short on time, rather than applying a highlight, contour, and midtone shade as usual, just sweep your midtone color across your eyelids for very subtle definition. It will help your eye color pop but won't help to define or shape your eyelids as much as using all three shades will.

You can also use a blush for your midtone, if the product has been approved for use near the eyes.

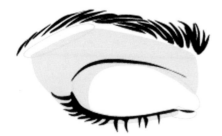

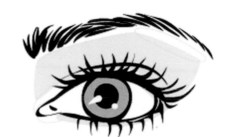

contour

Your contour shade is the deepest of the three shades. It's not necessarily stark or dark—it can even be metallic—but it is the deepest color. The contour eyeshadow is the shade you can have fun with and change with your mood. You'll find that most makeup lines offer more contour colors than highlight and midtone shades, because they are the most eye-catching and exciting to use. Because of its depth, your contour shade provides the most dramatic reshaping of your eyelid. This shade really helps define the eyes.

To apply, move a brush with shadow across your top lash line, from the outside corner toward the inside corner (brushing shadow along your lash line helps create a blended effect with your eyeliner, which is always more flattering and more youthful). Then, bring the color up into the outer portion of the crease and blend it inward (about a third or, at most, halfway across). Your goal is to create a gradation of color, with the outer corner of the eye being the darkest and becoming lighter as you move in toward the center of the eyelid. By layering your contour shade on top of your midtone shade, you'll get the blended, defined look you want. You can also apply the contour color underneath and along the lower lash line to define your eyes. (Blending it over your eye pencil gives it a softer, more subtle lined effect.) Visit page 56 to find the perfect shape brushes.

For a more dramatic eye, apply several layers of color, to build the shade's intensity. Add color in small amounts. You can always add more for extra drama, but once you've applied it, it's difficult to remove. If you need to soften your application, simply take a little loose powder and a clean brush, and blend it over the shadow you just applied. To soften your application, use a clean brush to apply a little loose powder over the shadow.

tips:

The first place you lay your brush will receive the most color, because it has the most eyeshadow on it at that point.

Because blending is so vital to the overall effect of beautifully painted eyes, good-quality shadow brushes are a must. Good brushes enable you to create artful shapes and effects.

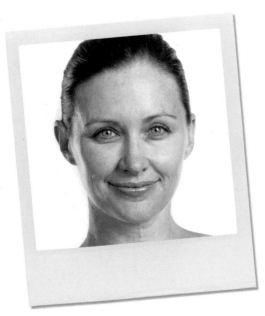

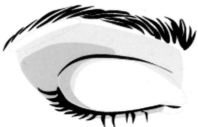

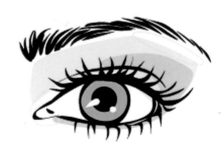

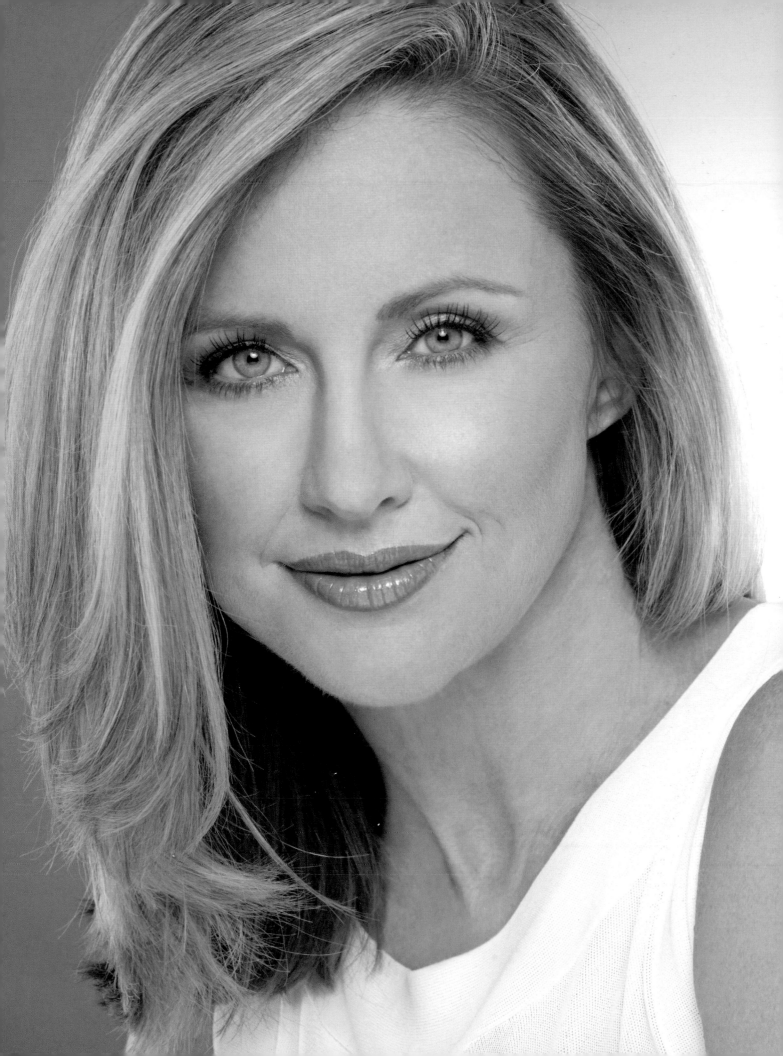

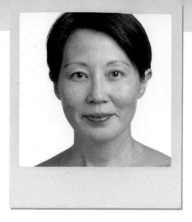

other eye shapes

hooded eyes

Hooded eyes are sometimes called "bedroom eyes," because the lids tend to look heavy and partly closed. There are two types of hooded eyes—those that you are born with and those that you acquire. Applied correctly, eye color can help hooded eyes appear more open by minimizing the eyelid.

- Avoid using a dark eyeshadow over the entire lid, because it can make the lid appear heavier and will make your eyes look closed and small.

- Don't be tempted to highlight the brow bone too much; this can accentuate the hooded appearance of the eyelid.

- Avoid applying your highlight shade over the entire lid; it will just make your lid look even more hooded.

application

1. **highlight shade:** Apply to brow bone and along the upper lash line. Also apply to the inside corner of the lower lash line.

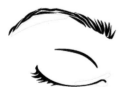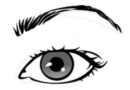

2. **midtone shade:** Start at the outside corner base of your upper lash line and bring the color up and over the entire hooded area. This helps the lid recede, by pushing the lid away and bringing the eye forward. Be sure to blend the areas where the midtone color meets the highlight color. Be sure to apply your midtone along your lower lash line; start from the outside corner and brush across toward the inside corner.

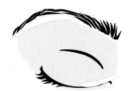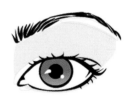

3. **contour shade:** Start at the base of the lash line and bring the color up and over the hooded area, layering it on top of your midtone. Do not bring it as far across as you did your midtone, but definitely come half way across the lid. Next, sweep your contour color underneath the lower lashes to define the lower lash line, starting from the outside corner and blending your way across. Don't miss this step! Hooded eyes really benefit from well-defined upper and lower lash lines.

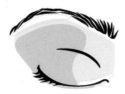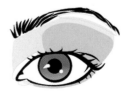

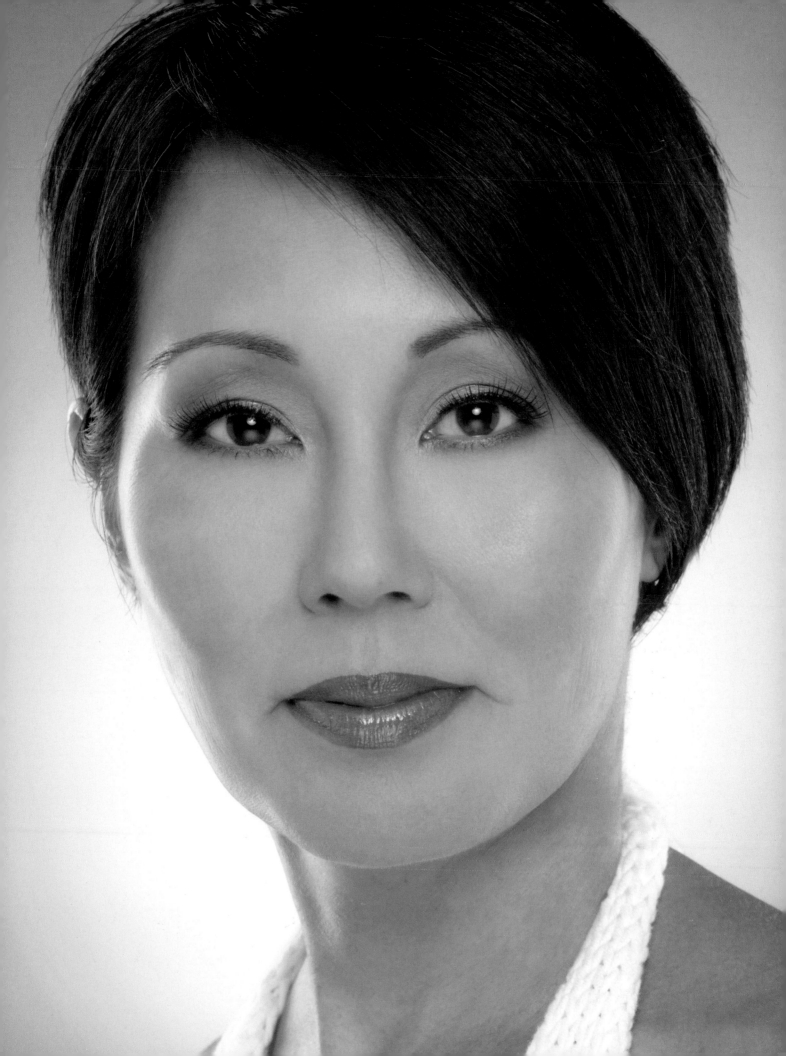

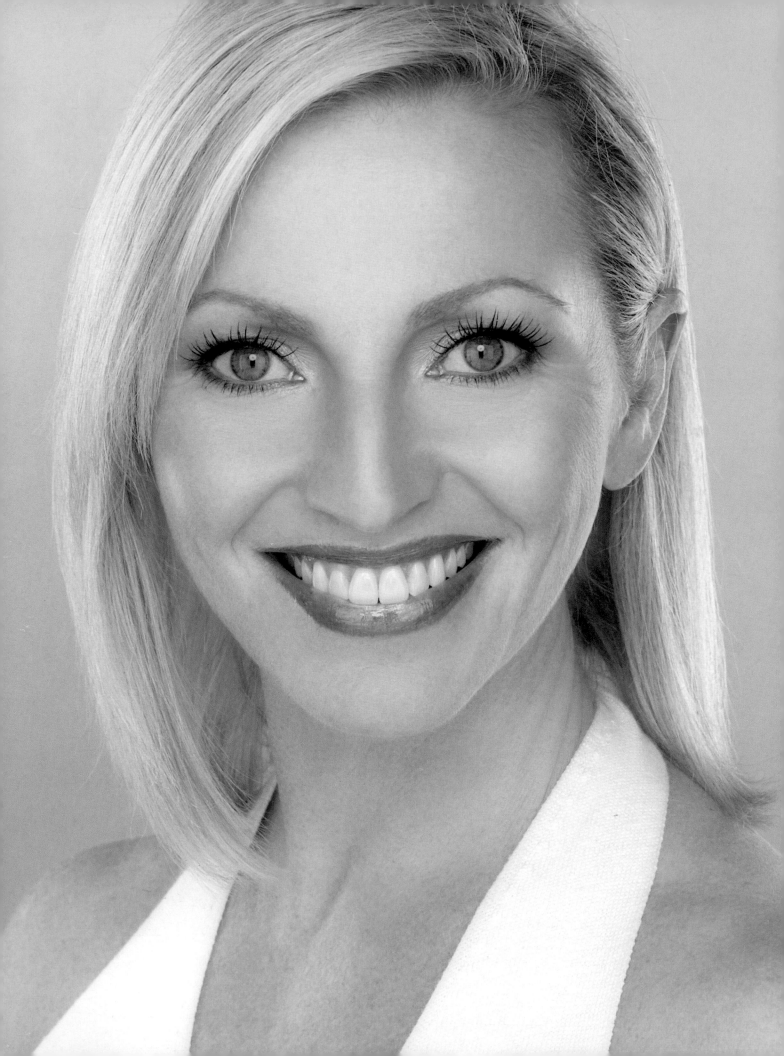

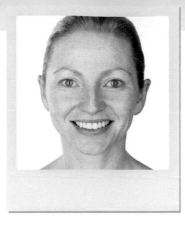

wide-set eyes

To determine whether or not you have wide-set eyes, measure the width of one eye. The space between your eyes should equal the width of one eye. If the space between your eyes is greater than one eye-width, your eyes are considered wide-set. Your goal is to create the illusion that they are set closer together (visually pushing them in).

- To visually "push" your eyes closer together, you need to darken the inside hollows of your eye next to the bridge of your nose. Deepening the color in this area helps your eyes appear to be set closer together. To get the needed color depth, do not bring your contour color all the way in—just layer your midtone shade.

- Begin any dark-color application slightly in from the outer corner of your eye and blend your shadow up and in instead of outward, because blending it outward will "pull" the eyes wider apart, and your goal here is to "push" them closer together.

application

1. **highlight shade:** Apply to your brow bone and eyelid.

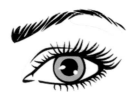
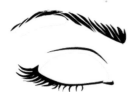

2. **midtone shade:** Starting from the outside corner of the crease, bring the color toward the inside corner of your eye, making sure to bring it up and in, not elongating it out. Be sure to apply a few extra layers to the inside corners, to deepen the color and help visually push the eyes closer together. Now apply your midtone along your lower lash line, starting from the outside corner and brushing across toward the inside corner. This helps start your definition and creates a better blend when you apply your contour shade and eyeliner.

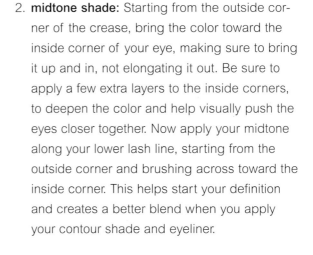
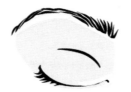
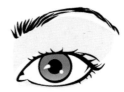

3. **contour shade:** Starting slightly in from the outer corner, brush it across the upper lash line and up into the crease of your eye. Also sweep it underneath the lower lash line, being careful not to extend the color beyond the outer edge of the eye.

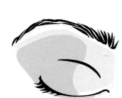
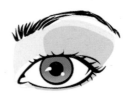

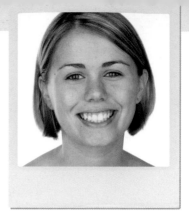

close-set eyes

The ideal space between your eyes should be approximately the width of one eye. If the space between your eyes is less than one eye-width, you have close-set eyes. Your goal is to create the illusion that your eyes are farther apart.

- Keep the inside corners of your eyes and the areas closest to your nose as light as possible, to help visually push the eyes apart.

- Concentrate the darker shades on the outer corners of your eyes. Always elongate your darkest shadows, to help pull the eyes apart.

application

1. **highlight shade:** Apply to your eyelid and brow bone. Also apply your highlight shade to the inside corner of the lower lash line. This helps to open up your eyes, making them appear larger and more youthful. This step is imperative for close-set eyes, because it really helps visually push the eyes apart.

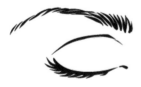

2. **midtone shade:** Starting at the outside corner of the crease, bring the color in toward the inside corner. With all other eye shapes, we have applied our midtone shade from the outside corner of the crease to the inside corner;

for close-set eyes, we will only bring it three-quarters of the way across, because we do not want to deepen the inside corner of the lid. This visually pushes the eyes closer together. We want to keep the area closest to the bridge of your nose as light as possible. Apply your midtone along your lower lash line, starting from the outside corner and brushing toward the inside corner. This helps to start your definition and create a better blend when you apply your contour shade and eyeliner.

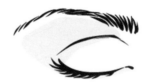

3. **contour shade:** Sweep it across the base of the upper lash line and up into the outer area of the crease. You definitely want to elongate this shade, to help pull the eyes apart. Confine it to the outer corners of the eyes—never bring it more than a third of the way in. Sweep it underneath the lower lash line for definition.

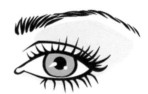

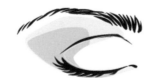
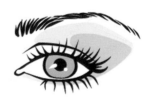

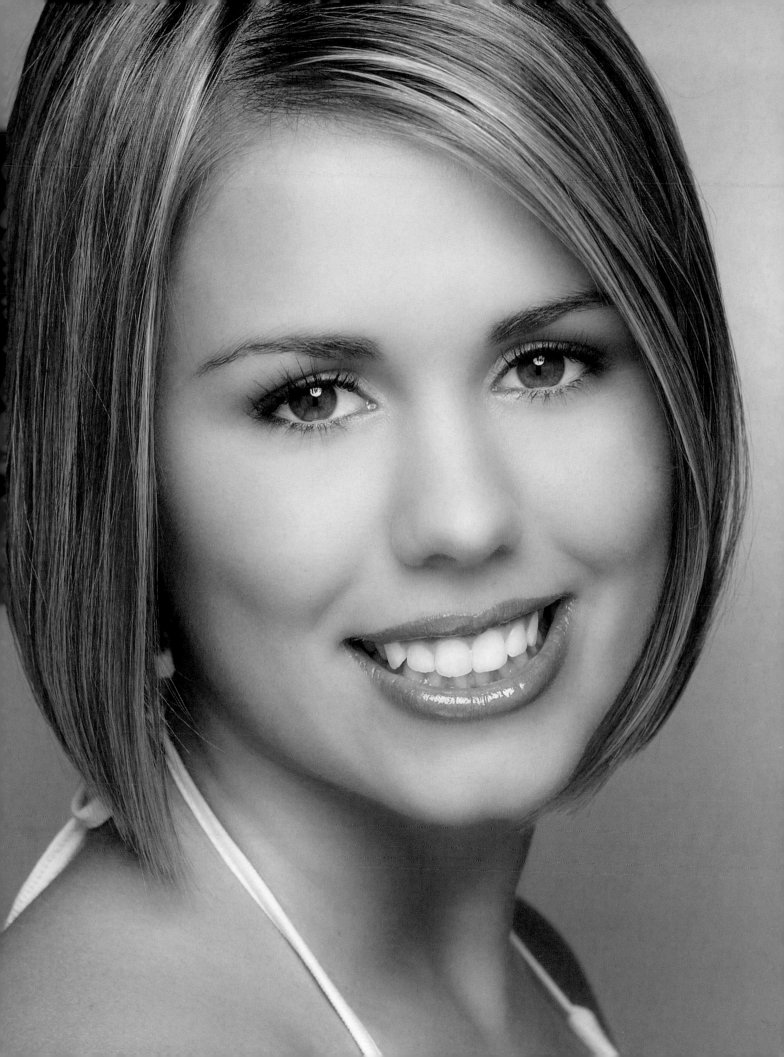

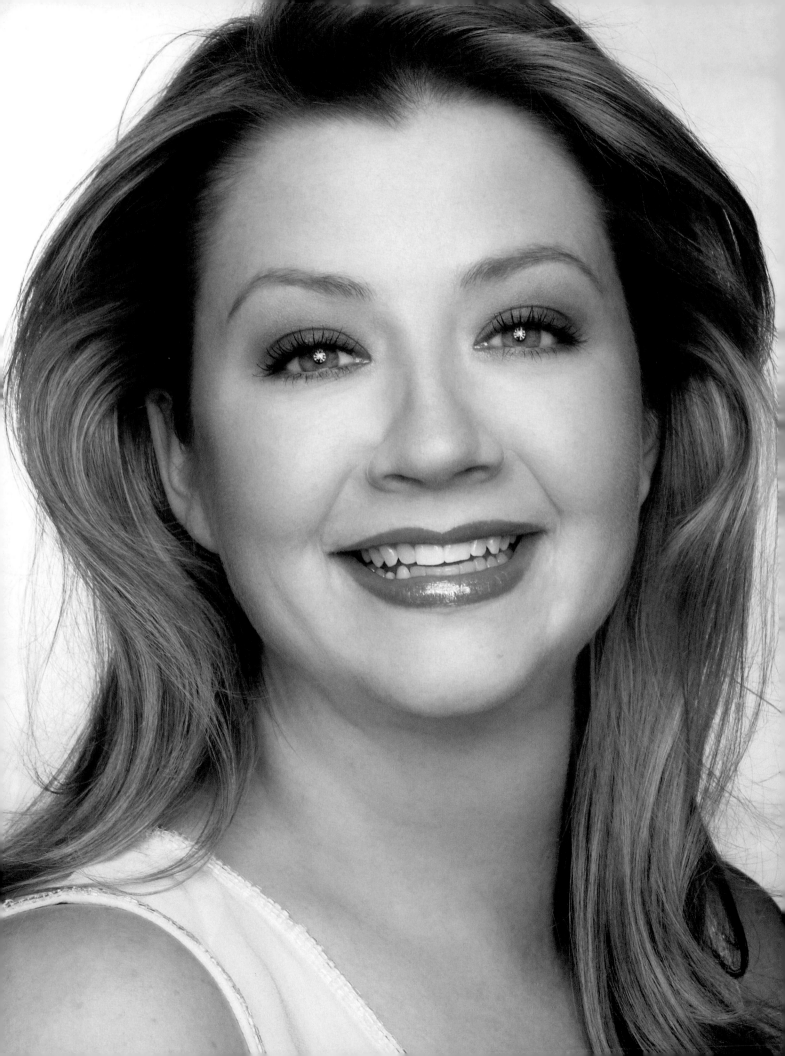

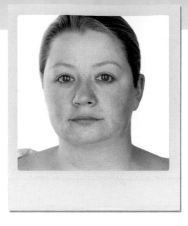

prominent eyes

If your eyelids and eyes are full and tend to extend out from the face, you have prominent eyes. The goal here is to visually push the eye away from us and help the eye appear to recede into the face. We do this by creating a light-to-dark effect with the three eyeshadows, with the darkest shade applied closest to the lash line and fading as you go toward the brow. For prominent eyes, we are actually trying to make the eyes appear smaller; we want to minimize their fullness.

- Never highlight your eyelids—your eyes will appear even more prominent. Remember, everything we highlight is visually pulled forward.

- A deeper or contour shade across the entire eyelid helps to minimize the fullness and makes it appear to recede.

- With this eye shape, you can apply your eyeliner all the way around your eye with the same thickness and intensity, because we actually want to close the eye in slightly.

application

1. **highlight shade:** Apply to brow bone only.

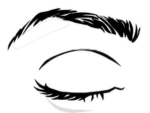

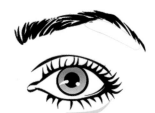

2. **midtone shade:** Start at the base of your upper lash line and bring the color up and over your entire lid, all the way up to your brow bone. Laying your brush first along your lash line and working your way upward gives you the highest concentration of color at the lash line. Be sure to apply your midtone along your lower lash line, starting from the outside corner and brushing across toward the inside corner. This helps start your definition and creates a better blend when you apply your contour shade and eyeliner.

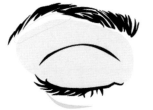

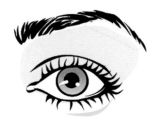

3. **contour shade:** Again, start at the base of your lash line and bring the color all the way across the lid and up into the crease. Then sweep the contour color underneath the lower lash line, to create definition and further help your eyes recede into your face.

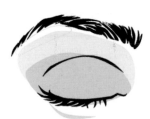

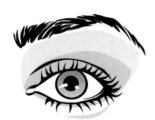

the eyes have it | 181

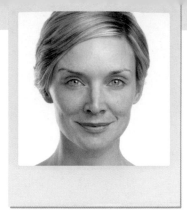

deep-set eyes

As the name suggests, deep-set eyes are eyes that are set deep into their sockets. The brow bone also extends out farther with this eye shape than with any other eye shape. The goal with deep-set eyes is to bring your eyes out and forward, while pushing your brow bone back, to make the eyes look more properly set on the face. The great thing about deep-set eyes is that they are much less likely to start to droop as you age.

- A dark eyelid does not work for this eye shape. You want to highlight the eyelids of deep-set eyes as much as possible, to help bring them out. A dark lid pushes them farther back into the head.

- Darkening the crease is also unnecessary for this eye shape. God has given you a crease, so there's no need to emphasize it.

- There is no need to highlight the brow bone, since it is already prominent. Highlighting brings it forward even more, and we want it to recede.

- When you wear eyeliner, keep it as close to the lash line as possible (very thin). Thick eyeliner, especially on the upper lids, will work against you when you're trying to bring out the eyes.

application

1. **highlight shade:** Apply to the eyelid and into the crease. This helps pull the eye forward. Also apply your highlight shade to the inside corner of the lower lash line.

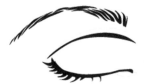 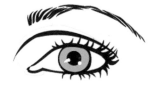

2. **midtone shade:** Apply your color right above the crease, not in the crease. Starting from the outside corner, bring it across the lid toward the inside corner just above the crease, blending it up onto the brow bone. Now, apply your midtone along your lower lash line, starting from the outside corner and brushing across toward the inside corner.

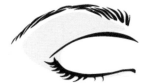 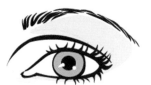

3. **contour shade:** Apply contour from the outer corner of the upper lash line, then up onto the brow bone, once again to help make the area recede. Next, sweep the contour color underneath the lower lashes to define the lower lash line, starting from the outside corner and blending your way across.

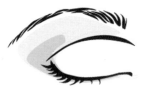 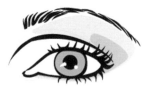

tip:

For drama, I always use a brighter (not necessarily a darker) color of shadow. This also keeps you from deepening your lid too much.

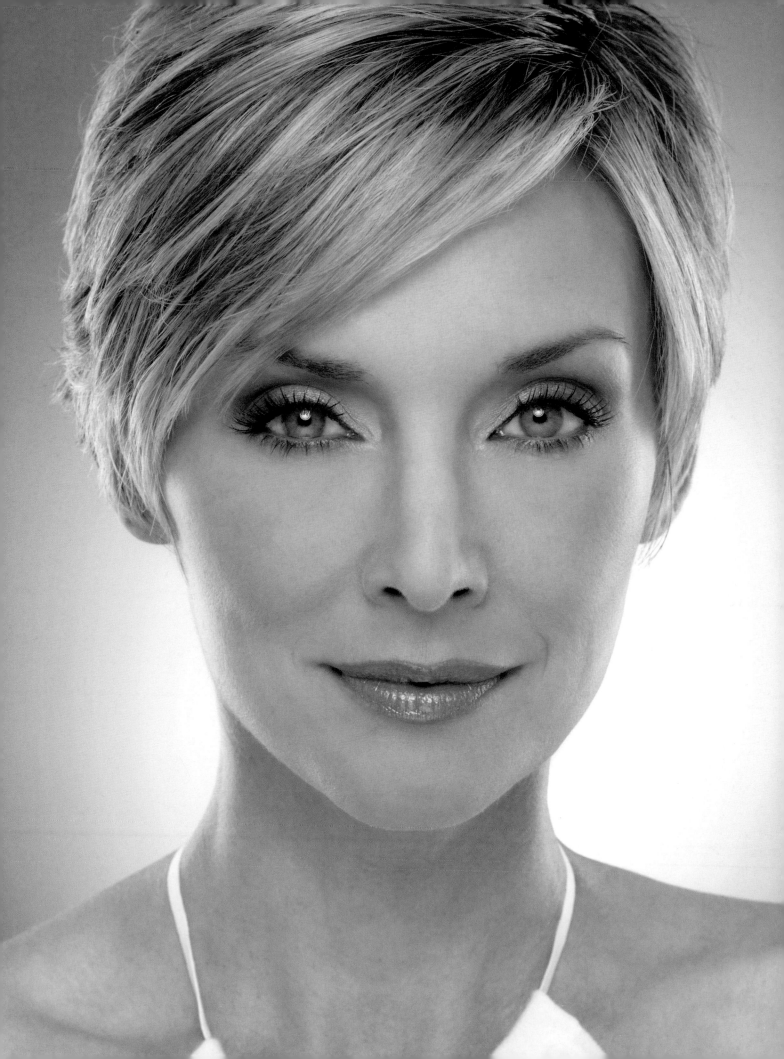

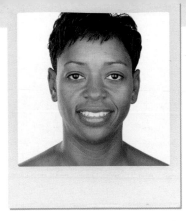

droopy eyes

By "droopy eyes," I do not mean that the lid is droopy; I mean that the outer corners of your eyes turn slightly downward. They are sometimes referred to as "sad, puppy-dog eyes." Your goal is to make the outer corners appear to turn up, rather than down. It's actually very easy to do! You just need to start your color application slightly in from the outside corner, on top and especially along the bottom lash line.

- You want to create what we call an "open-ended" eye, which means that the color from your top lash line and bottom lash line do not meet at the outer corner of the eye. If the color meets at the outside corner, it will accentuate the droop. By leaving it natural, you actually create a visual lift to the eye.

- When applying mascara, be sure to concentrate on the middle to inside lashes. Defined lashes in the outer corners of the eyes also accentuate the droopiness.

tips:

When wearing color along the lower lash line, begin your application about an eighth of an inch in from the outermost corner.

For this eye shape, I suggest not using eyeliner along the lower lash line. It can look too dramatic. Instead, use your contour shade to define along your lower lash line.

application

1. **highlight shade:** Apply to brow bone and eyelid. Also apply your highlight shade to the inside corner of the lower lash line.

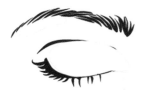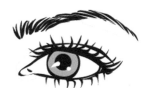

2. **midtone shade:** Starting slightly in from the outside corner of the eye, bring the color across and into the inside corner of the crease. Be sure to bring the color up and in. Now, starting just slightly in from the outer corner, apply your midtone along your lower lash line. Be sure to start from the outside corner and brush across toward the inside corner.

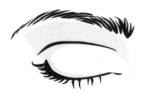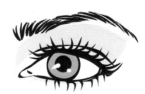

3. **contour shade:** Starting just slightly in from the outside corner, bring your color up and into the crease. Next, sweep contour color along the lower lash line, being sure once again to start slightly in from the outside corner.

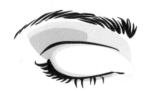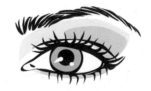

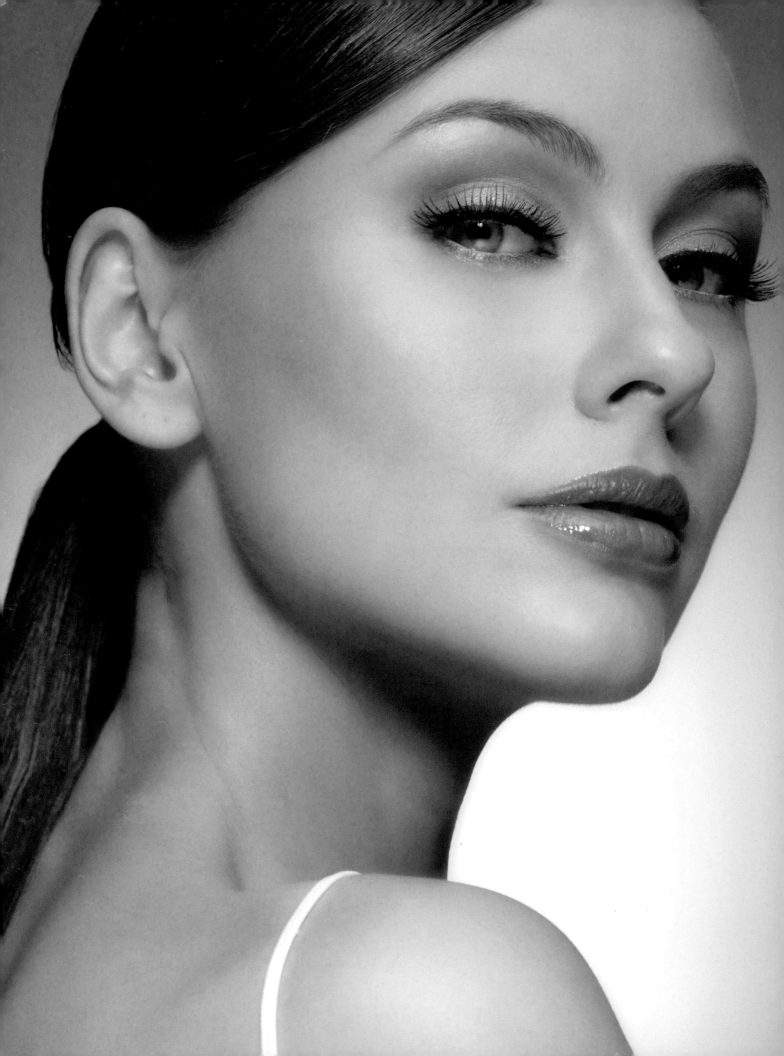

eyeliner

Eyeliner can go a long way toward helping to define your eyes (opening them up and drawing attention to them), but if used incorrectly, it can be very aging. One really important thing to remember is that to look your most youthful, you might want to soften your eyeliner color choice. Some women think they have to stop wearing eyeliner as they age, but that's just not true. They just need to make better color choices. For example, if you wore black eyeliner in your twenties, switch to brown, to create a softer, more youthful definition in your fifties. If you now think brown is too intense, switch to a soft bronze or taupe. Don't stop defining your eyes as you age, just soften the definition.

There are a number of ways to define your eyes when lining, but of course I will start with my personal preference. Over the years, I have discovered that it works best, while still looking soft and natural. But first, here are some ground rules:

- If you line along your bottom lash line, you *must* line across the top lash line. Without the balance along the top lash line, the depth along the bottom will pull the eye down and make them look older and tired.

- Likewise, the color along your bottom lash line should never be deeper than the color along your top lash line, because, this, too, will drag your eye down. Many women want more definition along the top lash line than along the bottom, and this is always okay. For example, a deep brown eyeliner along your top lash line with a soft bronze along the bottom creates a softer, more subtle look.

- You can line along the top lash line without lining along the bottom. I usually like a little definition along the bottom, even if it is just a little of your eyeshadow contour color. But you don't have to define along the bottom lash line.

- For a soft, natural look, you can skip eyeliner. But you can also get a natural look by using an eyeliner brush and a dark eyeshadow to add a little soft definition at your lash line. Using an eyeshadow instead of actual eyeliner gives you subtle definition, without making your eyes looked lined.

Although there are many lining options, your goal is always the same: to create definition and make the eyes the focus of your look. Even as you age, you still want to define your eyes; defined eyes wake your face up and create a wide-eyed, youthful expression. I am constantly asked where to apply the color. How far in do you go with the color? Where do you start, and where do you stop? Where should you line? How thick a line should you create?

There is a simple rule of thumb that works for all eye shapes. Along your top lash line, you want your definition to start at the inside corner of your eye. Here, the liner should be thinnest, then slowly make it become wider as you apply it across to the outside corner of the eye. This creates the definition that you are looking for without closing in the eye. Along your lower lash line, the color should be most intense at the outside corner, fading away as you move toward the inside corner. You want to bring it all the way across the bottom lash line, but make sure the color fades in intensity from the outer corner to the inner corner. The same thickness all the way across the top and underneath the lower lash line can close in your eyes and make them appear smaller, whereas a gradation of color across the top and along the bottom adds definition and attention. Place your color as close to the lash line as possible. You do not want skin showing between your lashes and your eyeliner!

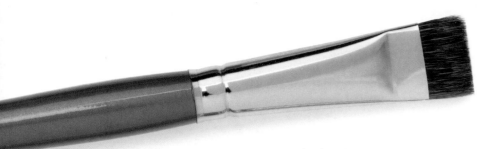

Let's talk about application options. Most often, I choose to line or create my definition around the eye with nothing more than the correct brush and a dark eyeshadow. Eyeshadow is not only the easiest to apply, it also creates the most subtle effect.

powder

1. Dip a dry eyeliner brush (refer to page 57 to see which shape works best for the effect you want to create) into your powder eyeshadow and tap off the excess.

2. Place your brush at the outside corner of the top lash line and sweep it toward the inside corner. This creates a subtle wash of color along the lash line.

3. Now for your lower lash line. Dip your brush (refer to page 57 for the shape that works the best for application and blending along the lower lash line) into your shadow and tap off the excess.

4. Starting from the outside corner (because the first place we lay the brush receives the highest concentration of color), sweep the color along your lower lash line, all the way across. This creates a fading of color from the outer corner (the deepest) to the inner corner (the lightest).

pencil

Some women find it difficult to apply eyeliner pencil. Here are some tricks to make it easier:

1. Do not feel that you have to apply your eyeliner in one straight, perfect line. Begin at the outside corner of your lower lash line and draw small, feather-like strokes (dashes), connecting each one as you move toward the inside of the eye. Use the same trick on the upper lash line.

2. You can make eyeliner pencil look more exact by using an eyeliner brush to blend across the line you just created and make it look like one solid, connected, mistake-free line. I also suggest this professional technique: Before using your brush to blend, dip it in a little eyeshadow. This helps smudge the line and soften its appearance. You can use a shade of eyeshadow that matches your eyeliner, or you can choose a different shade, to change and customize your liner color.

tip:

The sharper the point on your pencil, the easier and more precise the application, so always sharpen before you apply.

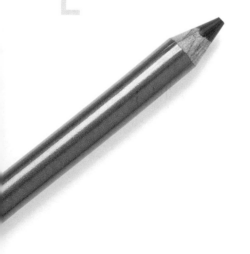

3. Once again, use your brush to blend the line. I find it especially effective to use an eyeshadow brush when blending. The outside corner—the first place you lay the brush—will receive the highest concentration of color, and sweeping your brush across blends the liner, helping it fade as you move inward. When you are finished, it will be darkest at the outside corner and lightest at the inside corner (creating the perfect fade), which, as you know, is your goal.

liquid, crème, and gel

These three types of eyeliner are all very similar in their appearance and application. They give you the most dramatic effect (think Audrey Hepburn and her signature cat-eyed eyeliner look). Because of this, they may not be your best choice if you are trying to look younger. If this is the form of eyeliner you like best though, here's a *looking younger* tip: Choose lighter shades. For example, instead of black, choose brown or bronze, so that it looks less harsh. One great advantage of liquid, crème, and gel eyeliners is that they usually have great staying power.

Use these eyeliners *only* along the top lash line. *Never* use them along the bottom lash line—they will look too harsh and stark and will never look natural. If you want color along your lower lash line, use pencil or powder for lower lash line definition. When applying these three formulas, practice definitely makes perfect.

How to apply them: Starting at the inside corner of your top lash line, move your applicator (liquid eyeliner comes with a brush or felt tip; for crème or gel, you will need an eyeliner brush) slowly across the lash line. Be sure to make your line its most narrow at the inside corner, gradually getting thicker as you reach the outside corner. As your brush reaches the outside corner, you can give it a little "kick" upwards, which helps lift the eye.

cake

This is a powder that looks much like an eyeshadow but is much heavier and more highly pigmented. Cake eyeliner is easy to apply and gives a similar effect to liquid, crème, or gel. Apply it in exactly the same way as you apply the other three, but dampen your brush before applying it. Be sure you use the right brush for the job (visit page 57 to help you figure out what type of brush you will need).

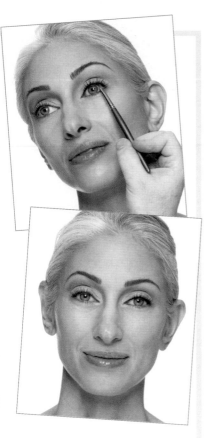

tip:

The professional secret to creating the perfect definition along the lash line is to get the color right into the base of the lashes (especially along the top lash line). There is a secret trick many of us makeup pros use to create definition like no other. Simply use a fine-tipped brush to carefully push black eyeshadow into the base of your eyelashes. This defines the eyes and makes your lashes look thicker, without making your eyes appear "lined." You can scrub a pencil into the base of your lashes, as well, but I find it easier to use eyeshadow and a brush. My brush #41 is perfect for this pro trick.

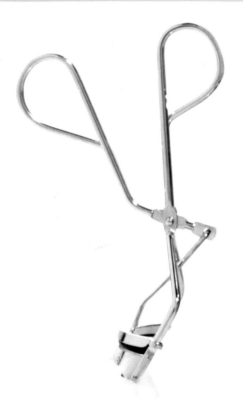

long lashes

I have five words to say about eyelashes: curl, curl, curl, curl, and curl. There is no quicker, cheaper, faster facelift than curling your eyelashes. It opens the eyes, lifts your lids, and makes you look years younger. If you don't think you need to curl, just look at the before and after pictures on the right to see what curling can do for you. All that our model has done is curl her lashes. You can see how much it has lifted her eye and made it appear more open, which translates to more youthful look. You are never too old to curl your lashes!

These days, you have many curling options and multiple tools to get the job done, including the classic crimp curler, a detailed, precision eyelash curler, and, one of my favorites, the heated eyelash curler (turn to page 60 to find your perfect tool). No matter which you choose, just remember you need to curl!

The classic crimp curler is fast and easy, but be sure the tool you use is fairly new. If you use an eyelash curler for more than a

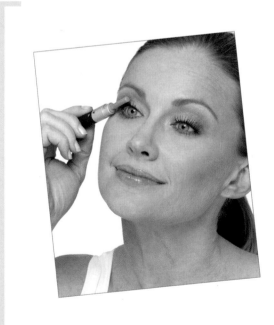

tip:

For those afraid of crimp-style eyelash curlers, there is now an alternative curling tool: a heated eyelash curler. This tool is used after you've applied mascara, a great feature, since many times when you apply your mascara after curling, it can slightly uncurl your lashes. To use, start at the base of your lashes and work the curler back and forth, from side to side at the base of your lashes, so that your lashes fall into the grooves of the curler. Now push up and twist the curler in toward your lid. Your lashes will be curled to perfection—no crimping needed!

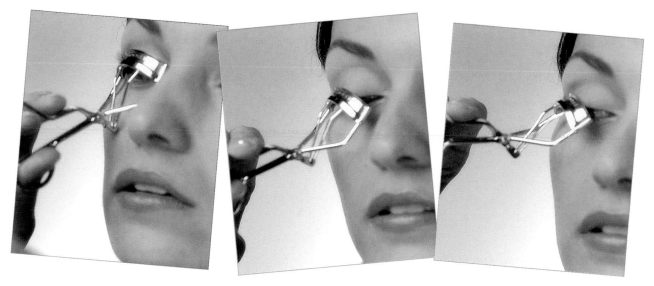

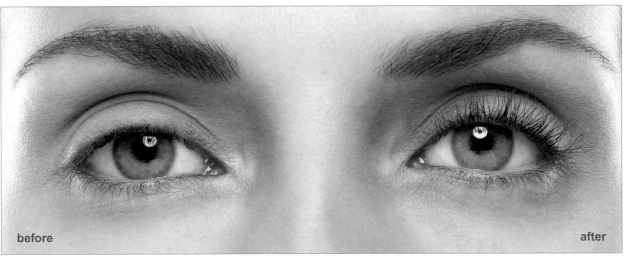

before   **after**

year, it can get out of alignment and cut your lashes. So, throw the one from high school out—it is time to buy a new one! You need to replace a crimp curler every year and change the rubber piece every six months.

The trick to curling your eyelashes correctly using a crimp curler is to crimp them more than just once at the lash line. Instead, "walk" the curler along the length of your lashes, taking care to close, open, and move the eyelash curler up, until you reach the end of your lashes. Depending on the length of their lashes, some women crimp once, some might crimp

three times; the point is to walk it out and crimp as many times as you can till you reach the end of your lashes. This method creates a curve, rather than a crimp and helps your eyelashes stay curled.

A detailed precision eyelash curler works the same way a classic crimp curler works. The difference is in its size—it is only one quarter as wide as the classic version, which makes it easier to get right to the base of the eyelashes. Start at the base of the lashes and crimp outward, to the ends of your lashes, just as you did with the classic crimp curler.

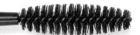

mascara

Mascara is everyone's favorite way to add definition to the eyes. I recommend applying several coats of mascara, to define and open your eyes, because layering your mascara creates the most dramatic definition. If you have allergies or are concerned about getting teary-eyed, you can make any formula waterproof by topping your regular mascara with a layer of waterproof mascara. Here's the best way to apply several coats of mascara to "build" lashes that last:

1. Begin by curling your eyelashes with a crimp-style curler; this opens up the eyes and makes them appear larger and more youthful. (If you opt for a heated curler, use it after you've applied your mascara and it has thoroughly dried.)

2. Pull the mascara wand out of the tube and wipe the brush against the opening of the tube or on a paper towel to remove excess product. Do not be afraid of cleaning too much product off—there is plenty on there!

3. Apply the small amount that is left on the brush to your eyelashes.

4. Using an eyelash comb, comb your lashes before the mascara dries. This will help keep your lashes well separated and prevent them from clumping.

5. Let each coat of mascara dry between applications. This can take a couple of minutes, so be patient, but each coat must be completely dry. If you do not wait for each layer to dry, your lashes will clump.

6. After one coat is dry, pull your wand out, clean it off, and apply your next coat. Comb, dry, and so on and so on—you get the picture.

The trick to mastering multiple-coat application is being sure to apply very thin coats, letting each dry completely between layers. I almost always apply three coats to the top lash line and one coat to the bottom.

There is no rule stating that you have to apply mascara to your bottom lashes; it is a matter of personal preference. When I first started my makeup career (many, many years ago), I would never use mascara on the bottom lashes (it was not in fashion), but now I almost always do (for definition). The one time I might try to convince you not to use mascara along your lower lash line is if your lashes are very sparse, because defining them only accentuates their sparseness.

Here's a *looking younger* trick of the trade: If you don't use mascara on your lashes, be sure to smudge your eyeliner really well, because mascara breaks up the line and makes it look much more natural. Remember that defining your eyes always makes your eyes look more youthful, which makes *you* look more youthful. I think that thick, dark, long lashes are eighty percent of the battle—your lashes are so important. Curled, thick, dark, luscious lashes equals young and beautiful.

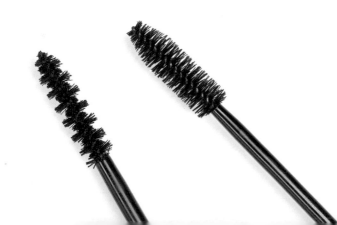

Now, we come to the ever-present question of color: black versus brown versus a color (such as blue or purple, for example). I feel very strongly about mascara color, because your eyelashes are so important in giving your eyes definition. For me, the answer is always black, because if I am going to have a party, I am going to have a big one! Black gives you the most definition. I am not opposed to brown or black/brown, especially if these shades make you feel more comfortable. Choose one of these colors if you want a softer result (less definition). Colored mascara is always a *no* for me; it does *not* look natural and does nothing for your eyes. Stay away! The more defined your eyes, the more youthful you will appear.

It's important to choose the correct formula of mascara for your desired effect. If you just want to define your eyelashes, use a defining formula. If you want to thicken and lengthen your lashes, choose a formula that will build them. Thickening and lengthening mascaras contain small particles that attach to the lash to add bulk and length. (Turn to page 40 for more information on mascara formulas.) I think every woman should want long, thick lashes. But ultimately, you'll control whether or not your lashes appear longer and thicker through the application technique you choose.

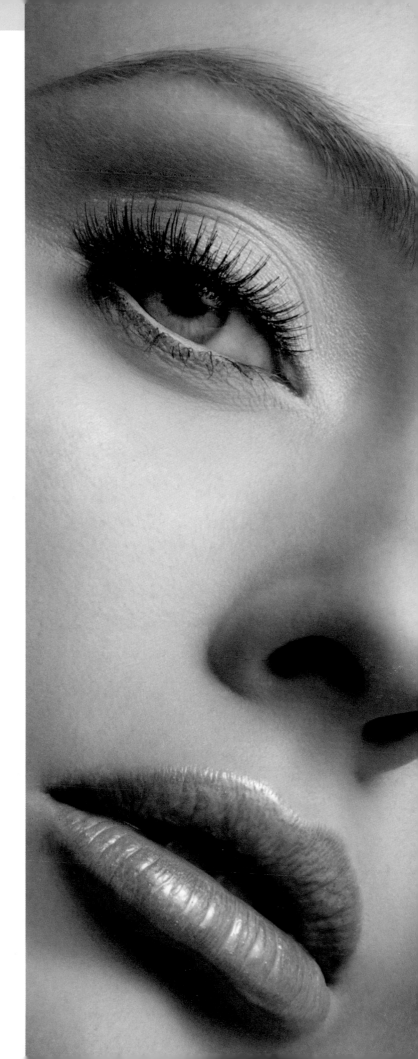

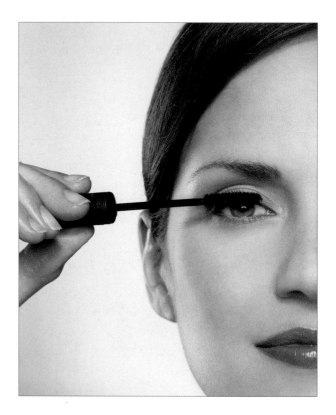

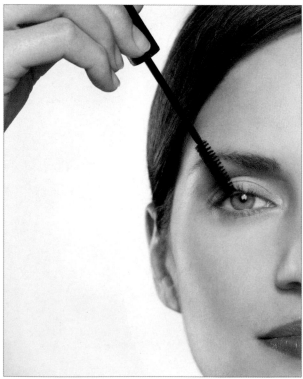

For thicker lashes: Start at the base of the lashes and hold your mascara wand in a horizontal position, working it from side to side, as you work your way up to the end of the lashes. The mascara particles will attach to the sides of your lashes and make them appear thicker.

For longer lashes: Hold your mascara wand in a vertical position. Starting at the base of the lash line, pull the wand up and out to the end of your lashes. The particles will attach to the ends of your lashes, making them appear longer.

If you want both—and you deserve both—simply apply multiple layers, using both techniques. For example, apply your thickening coat (horizontally), then let it dry. Then apply your lengthening coat (vertically) and let it dry, and so on. Don't forget: If you want to waterproof your lashes, use waterproof mascara for your final layer.

Be sure to choose the correct formula for your desired effect. If you want to define your lashes, use a defining formula. If you want to thicken them, use a thickening formula. (Turn to page 40 for more information on the different mascara formulas available.) If you want your mascara to lengthen your lashes and don't use a lengthening formula, you will never achieve the results you want, because it won't have the tiny particles that adhere to the ends of your lashes and make them look longer. Buying the right formula for your needs will save you worlds of grief.

Q&A

My mascara always seems to smear and smudge, even if I wear a waterproof variety. What can I do to keep my mascara from smudging and smearing?

If your mascara smudges and smears, even with a waterproof formula, chances are, the mascara is not adhering to your lashes. There are a couple of things to try: First, you have to powder (with loose or pressed powder) under your eyes, to set your foundation and concealer. Not setting the two can cause your mascara to smear. Second, you need to make sure the mascara can grab onto your lashes. When you apply moisturizer and eye crèmes, avoid getting them on your lashes (it's very easy to accidentally do). If you do, the mascara can't adhere to your lashes, and it will smudge and smear.

My favorite mascara does not come in a waterproof formula, and I need it to be more water-resistant. I find waterproof formulas harder to remove, so I am not sure I want it to be waterproof, and I love the way my current formula builds. What are my options? Is there anything that I can do?

You absolutely can fix this problem! You can create custom effects by simply layering different mascara formulas. If you want your mascara to be more water-resistant, simply apply a layer of a waterproof formula after you use your current favorite mascara. You'll get the building effect you like (or whatever you like about your current favorite), with the advantage of waterproofing. The waterproof formula will also be easier to remove, because it is not directly on your lashes. You can customize your mascara effect by layering different mascara formulas; just be sure to let each layer dry between each coat.

tips:

I always find that, when I pull a mascara wand out of its tube, it has more product on it than I want (especially because I like to layer), regardless of the formula. Be sure to clean the excess off your brush before you apply mascara.

Be certain to coat your lashes with mascara at the inner and the very outer corners of your eyes. These are two areas that many women miss.

Two or three thinly applied coats of mascara are far more effective than a single clumpy one.

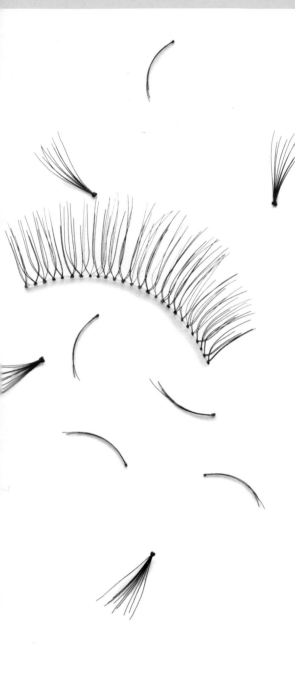

false eyelashes

If you really want to draw attention to your eyes, or if your natural lashes are thinning with age, you can always wear false eyelashes. They can be fun to play with for a special occasion or a special night out. Use false eyelashes, instead of depending on heavy eyeliner and overly intense eyeshadow, to define the eyes at the lash line, when you want more drama.

False eyelashes are available in strips, individual flares, and single strands. Strip lashes are the most commonly used and are readily available. I know that applying false eyelashes can seem intimidating, so here is an easy, foolproof way to apply strip false eyelashes. Regardless of your makeup IQ, this application technique will work for you and look natural. Just follow these easy steps to false eyelash perfection:

1. Curl your natural eyelashes. If your natural lashes grow straight out and down and you don't curl them, the false lash will also lie straight out and down. Definitely not our goal, so curl first.

2. Lay a mirror on the table or counter in front of you and look down. This puts your lid in the perfect position; you can see what you're doing, and you'll be much more comfortable waiting for everything to dry in this position than you would be if you were holding your chin up and looking into a wall mirror.

3. Draw a thin line across your upper eyelid right along your lash line with a black eyeliner pencil. This helps you to see where to place the lash and also helps conceal the lash band. Also, if you don't get the false lash in place directly against your natural lashes, no one will know, because the liner assures that no skin shows between your natural lashes and the false ones.

4. Trim the outside end of your false eyelashes to fit the width of your eyelid. Strip lashes are usually too wide for most eyes. Trimming them will help them fit better and feel more comfortable.

5. Apply eyelash glue along the false eyelash band. Allow the glue to dry for a minute, so it becomes tacky (slightly sticky), then place the lash right on top of your eyeliner. Using the handle end of a pair of tweezers, push the lash right up against your natural lash line.

6. Once the glue has dried, apply a coat of mascara, to blend your natural lashes with the false ones.

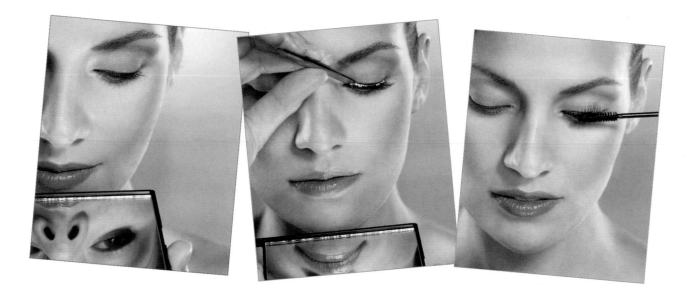

Want to wear false eyelashes, but want the look to be more natural than a strip? Individual flares and single strands look much more natural but still demand attention. Individual flares and single strands are a breeze to apply. Here's how:

1. Curl your natural eyelashes. If your natural lashes grow straight out and down and you don't curl them, the false lash will also lie straight out and down.

2. Lay a mirror on the table or counter in front of you and look down. This puts your lid in the perfect position, you can see what you're doing, and you'll be more comfortable than if you are holding your chin up and looking into a wall mirror, while everything dries out.

3. Apply a layer of mascara to give your natural lashes more bulk and make it easier to attach the false lashes.

4. Squeeze a dot of lash adhesive onto the lash packaging. This way, you can just dip your lash into the glue. Using a pair of tweezers, grab a flare or single strand. Now dip the root end into the adhesive.

5. With adhesive on the end of the lash, lay it right on top of one of your own lashes, with the root of the false lash as close as possible to your natural root. Continue all across your lash line, one flare or strand at a time.

6. When the adhesive has dried, apply another coat of mascara, to blend everything together.

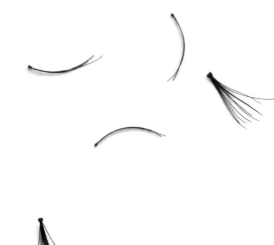

patty, 50s

What a spirit. Looking at Patty, I could feel her zest for life. I wanted to make her look as young as she felt inside. Defined eyes and beautiful, luscious lips did the job.

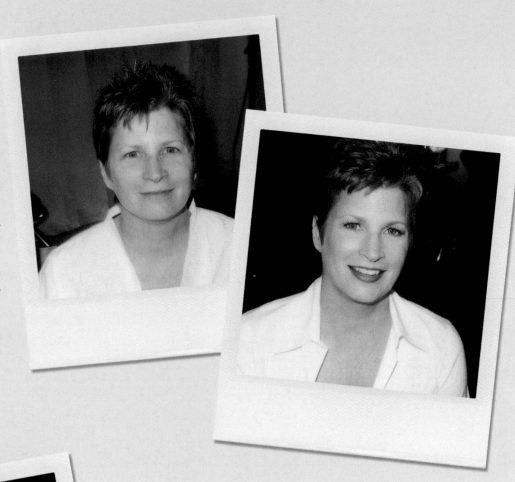

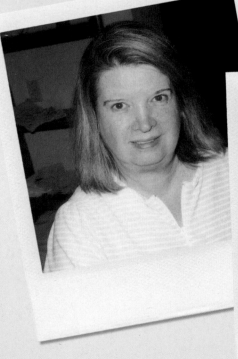

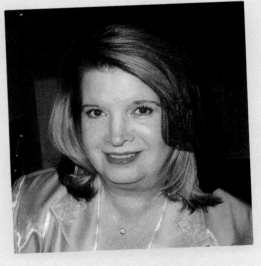

vikki, 50s

Talk about not looking your age! Vikki is a powerhouse. You can tell she makes things happen. It did not take much to make her look younger, just a little definition at the lash line and some beautiful color to her lips.

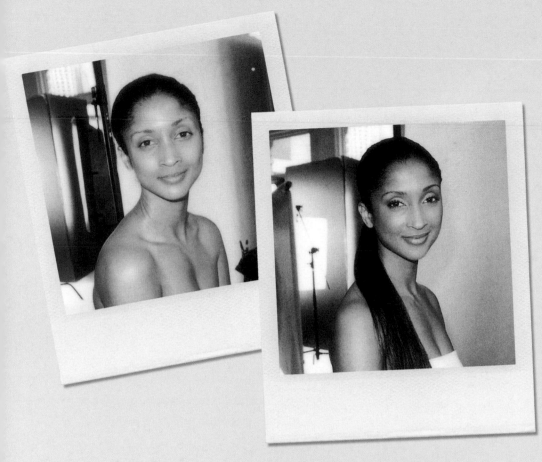

roshanda, 30s

All I could see was that Roshanda has a natural spark and light in her eyes. I love that I was able to take her natural strength and enhance those eyes. Unbelievable skin.

holly, 30s

Holly's coloring makes everything less than visible. I proved that giving the right definition to her eyes (curled lashes and multiple layers of mascara) can define them to perfection. What a difference.

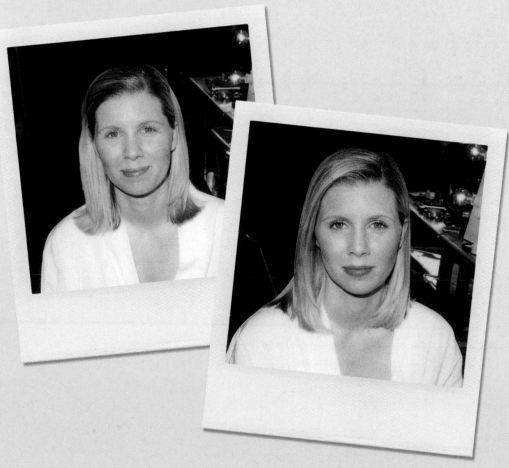

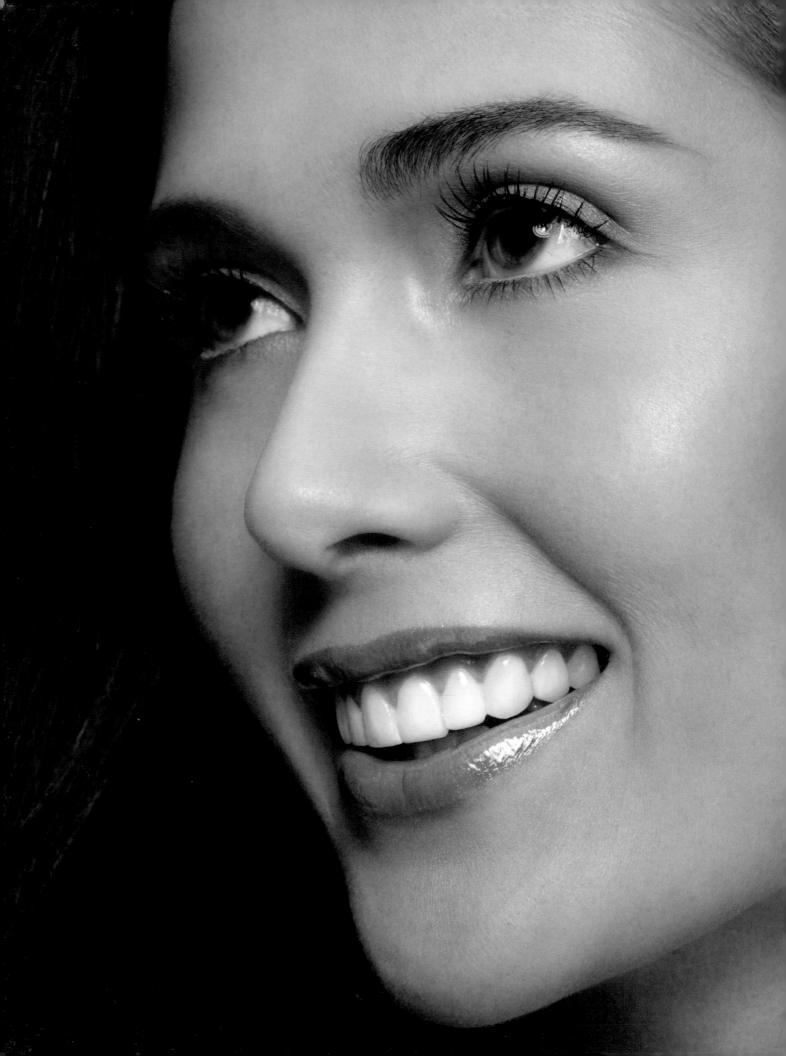

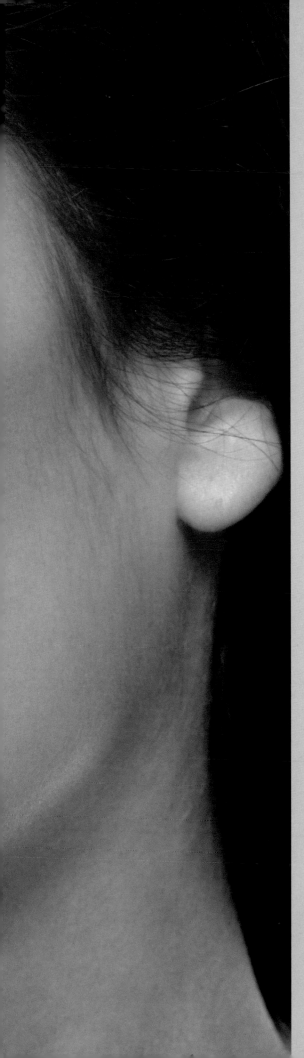

9

getting cheeky

I think one of the worst aspects of aging is losing color (depth) in your skin. It causes you to look pale and washed out—definitely not what I think of as youthful. But looking younger can be as simple as the sweep of a bronzer and blush brush (thank goodness!). Using the correct bronzer and blush is the most effective way to create that youthful glow I keep talking about. For me, bronzer and blush always go together; neither is as effective without the other. Every woman can benefit from a little bronzer! You are not necessarily trying to look like you just got back from St. Tropez—you just want to give your face a little color. And every woman looks younger with a slight flush to her cheeks—like you had a really good night, last night (even if you didn't). The combination of these two products is what creates the glow. There are two key factors to your success: choosing the right shades and proper placement. Let's talk color choices first.

bronzer

Our goal with bronzer is not to make you look like you have a tan; it's just to give the skin a youthful hint of color. For this reason, you want a bronzer that is one or two shades darker, not a great deal darker, than your skin. Women with ivory/beige skin tones will definitely want a shade of bronzer that is darker than their natural skin tone (but never more than two shades darker).

Now let's get more specific.

One of the most challenging aspects of picking out a bronzer is choosing the right shade. You do not want ivory/beige skin to be too orange, for example—there is nothing worse than a bright orange, overly bronzed face. Unfortunately, most of the products out there are too orange, so you'll need to be discerning when making your color choice.

For ivory skin, choose a bronzer with a neutral tone (flesh-colored, with a slight peach or pink tone to it). If you have beige skin, you can go for more of a golden tan undertone, which is perfect for your warm glow. For olive (darker beige) skin, a bronzer with a saturated terra-cotta or neutral brown undertone will give you the color you need. And for bronze/ebony skin, an intense copper or rich, warm brown works best. If you have dark ebony skin, keep in mind that your bronzer is not meant to deepen your skin color—you already have beautiful, rich depth to your skin—you just want to give your skin a glow. So, choose a bronzer that is darker than your skin tone, with a slight shimmer, to give you the glow you want.

Regardless of your color choice, keep in mind that bronzers with a matte finish will always look the most natural on ivory/beige skin. I always choose a matte finish for day, because its appearance is more natural. I might layer with a little shimmer over the matte shade, for a little extra glow at nighttime, but I always start with a matte bronzer first.

I also choose a bronzer with a matte finish for light bronze skin, because it gives the most natural effect. But darker bronze to ebony skin needs a little shimmer. If the finish is too matte, it can appear ashy on the skin. Don't go heavy on the shimmer, because it can be too much, even on dark skin. A light shimmer, however, can provide that youthful glow you are looking for.

Q&A **I have tried every shade of bronzer I can find, but they all look fake and too intense. You say I need one for a youthful glow. What are my options?**

If you feel that most bronzers are too heavily pigmented and give you more intense color than you want, try using a pressed powder instead. If you have ivory/beige skin, a bronze skin-tone pressed powder can work wonderfully as a bronzer. Powder contains fewer pigments, which helps it blend beautifully and look soft, subtle, and natural. You'll still get your youthful glow—it will just be toned down a notch.

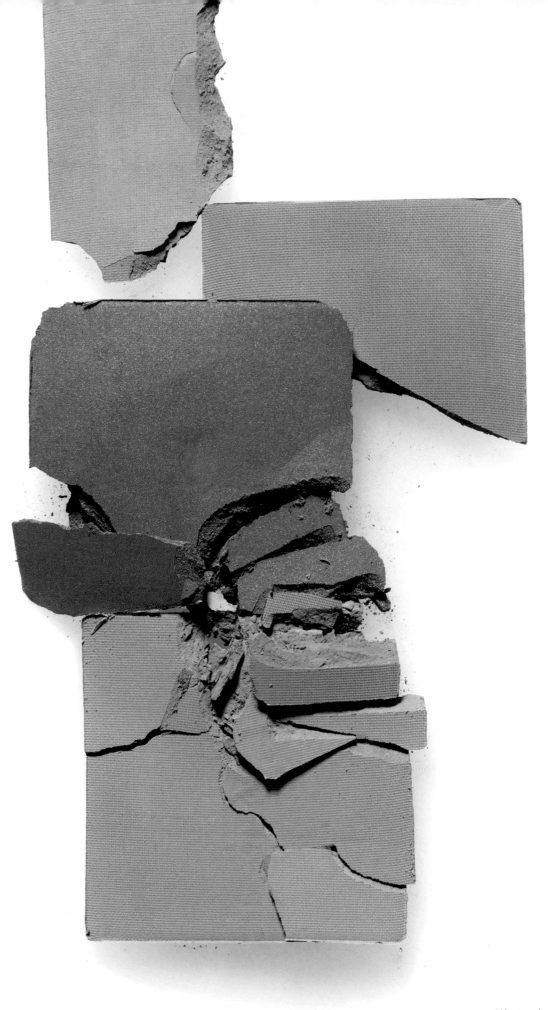

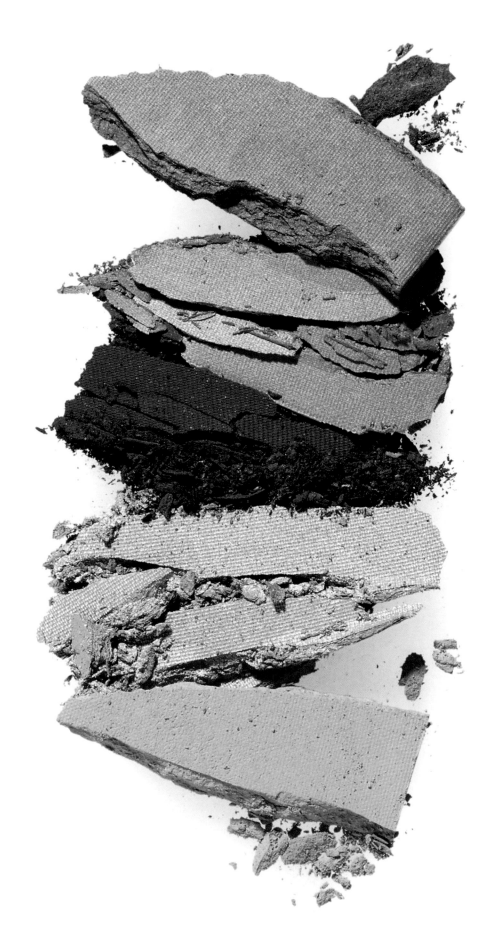

blush

I have to say, when it comes to choosing blush, many women make the wrong color choices, and looking younger is all about making the right color choice. The purpose of blush is to add color and life to the face. Blush is not used to contour or reshape the face (you should already have done that with foundation and powder; see page 127 to learn how). Avoid dark or heavy colors; you want a shade that is bright and fresh—youth in a neat little package.

Blush can brighten your face and make it positively glow. The trick is to find a blush color that's natural and neutral but still brightens and adds life to the skin. When determining your shade choice, a great place to start is to think about what shade your skin naturally flushes. Not sure what that is? Pinch your cheeks or jog around the block—this will give you a good idea. That shade is the depth you want, no darker. Dark, heavy shades will just age you, which is *not* our goal! We want young and pretty. Think bright, fresh, and young.

For ivory/beige skin tones, a blush with a soft peach or a warm pink undertone is the best choice. As you age, you want to definitely choose a blush with peach undertones, instead of pink, to help your skin appear brighter and fresher. Peach is a woman's best friend as she ages. It can warm and enhance the skin like nothing else, while pink often appears ashy and artificial on aging skin.

Women with olive skin tones (darker beige) should use blush with warm undertones and a richness or intensity, so the color shows up on the skin—tawny shades of dark coral or rich sienna, for example. If your skin tone is in the bronze/ebony category, you should also choose a blush with rich, intensely warm undertones, such as bright apricot or a warm brick, to give your skin a natural warm glow. For more drama and intensity, women with bronze/ebony skin tones (especially when the skin is dark ebony) can choose a blush with rich plum or red-brown undertones. The very best choice for all skin tones is a blush that looks soft and natural and appears to give you a glow from within.

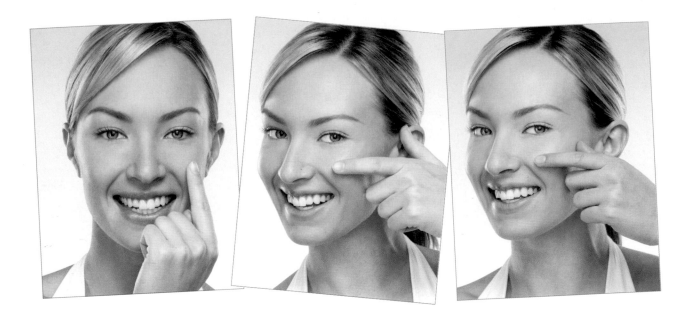

application

Many women are completely confused about how to apply their bronzer and blush, and because they are such important steps toward looking younger, I want to dispel some of the old myths about placement.

1. *Blush should never be worn closer to your nose than the width of two fingers.* Depending on the width of your fingers, your blush could wind up on the side of your face, instead of coming all the way to the apples of your cheeks! This rule clearly doesn't work for everyone.

2. *Blush should never be applied to your cheek below the tip of your nose.* If you have a cute little turned-up nose and you followed this advice, your blush could end up above the apples of your cheeks (on top of your cheekbones). So, this certainly doesn't work for everyone.

3. *Mature women should apply cheek color higher on the face as they age.* Although the skin may lose some of its elasticity as we age, I can assure you that our cheekbones remain in the same place! If you know how to locate your cheekbones correctly, you'll always have your bronzer and blush in the right place on your face.

Forget the old myths! Finding the right placement is easy. When applying bronzer and blush, you want to concentrate the majority of your color on the cheekbone; that is the proper placement. Where exactly is your cheekbone? No worries—it's easy to find. Just take this can't-miss application placement test:

1. Smile.
2. Locate the center of the apple of your cheek and place your index finger there.
3. Next, place your thumb at the top of your ear where it connects to your head.
4. Now take your thumb and bring it toward your index finger. The bone you feel is your cheekbone.
5. Apply your color directly onto the cheekbone.

tip:

Use separate brushes for your bronzer and blush. This prevents your colors from mixing and makes each color application clearer and more effective.

bronzer options

Bronzer makes your skin look sun-kissed and alive. It gives your skin a healthy glow without subjecting it to damaging ultraviolet rays. To warm your face and accentuate your bone structure, dust bronzing powder or crème bronzer along your cheekbones, the outer edges of your face, and your temples. Bronzer is also useful for lightly sculpting the nose and defining your jaw-line and chin. (See the Q&A on page 146 for more on this.)

powder

1. Be sure to use a nice, fluffy, full bronzer brush; this will help with your blending and give you the most natural application. Always apply your bronzer by beginning at the back of your cheekbone and sweeping it forward toward the apple of your cheek, then take the brush back toward your ear. This lays your color in place.

2. Now swipe your brush in the opposite direction (up and down) to blend. Be sure to blend well, so it looks natural.

3. Don't forget to add a little at the temples, to help shape your face. Sweeping the bronzing powder up around the temples and eye sockets can also really help your eye color pop, especially if your eyes are green or blue.

crème and gel

1. Use your finger or a sponge to dot color all along your cheekbone. Start at the apple of your cheek and work back toward your ear.

2. With a clean finger or sponge, blend the color out (up and down) and back toward your ear.

3. Go ahead and blend a little up onto your temples for the ultimate glow.

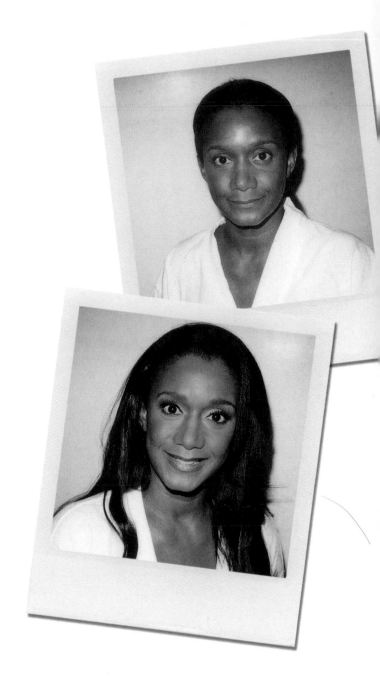

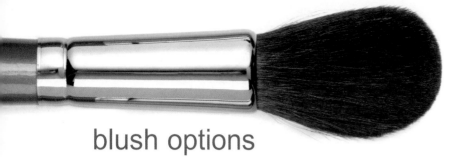

blush options

powder

Powder blush is the easiest to use. As with bronzer, you want to be sure you use a soft, full brush for the best application (it will help you achieve the most natural and blended look). You can apply your powder blush in two ways: one gives you more intense color, and the other gives you a soft, natural flush:

1. For the most color, apply blush to your cheekbone area, starting at the back (closest to your ear). Sweep the cheek color toward the apple of your cheek, then back toward the ear again. This lays your color in place.

2. Now, swipe your brush in the opposite direction (up and down) to blend. This way, your most intense color lies at the back of your cheek and gives your face more dimension.

3. For a soft flush of color, you can try a technique called "popping your apples." First, apply bronzer to your cheekbones (which I know you have already done, because you know how beneficial it is in our quest to look younger). Smile and apply a light, sheer, colorful blush (be sure it is not too dark) on the apples of your cheeks, blending back toward the bronzed area. This gives the apples of your cheeks a beautiful glow, because that is where you placed the highest concentration of color. Be sure to use a sheer shade of blush for this technique. A dark or intense cheek color can look too harsh and unnatural, when applied this way. Your goal is to glow, not to paint Raggedy Ann–style circles on your cheeks.

crème or liquid blush

If you use crème or liquid blush, apply it with a sponge or your fingers after your foundation and before your powder, for easier blending. If you wear blush without foundation, crème and liquid work better than powder blush, because they contain moisture that blends with the natural moisture of your skin. To apply crème or liquid blush, first dot a little onto the apples of your cheeks and then blend it back toward your ears.

With any blush, you should remember this rule: Always match textures—crème on crème and powder on powder. For example, you want to be sure to apply crème or liquid blush after your foundation and before you powder. If you wait until after you powder, it will not go on smoothly or evenly. Powder blush should be applied after your foundation and powder. If you try to apply it before you powder, it will go on splotchy and uneven.

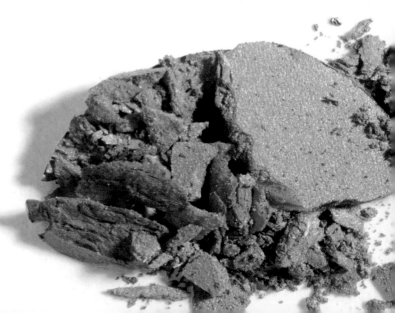

Q&A

I have tried everything: crème, powder, and liquid blush. Nothing stays on—my skin seems to absorb it all. What can I do to keep color on my face?

You can increase the wearability and intensity of your color by layering your blush. Layering blush textures helps the color last all day.

1. After applying your foundation, apply a crème blush to the apples of your cheeks and cheekbones.
2. Dust your face with loose or pressed powder.
3. Apply a powder blush (similar in color to the crème blush) to the apples of your cheeks and cheekbones.

I have very dry skin, and when I wear powder blush it seems to just sit on top of my skin. It never seems to look natural. What can I do?

For very dry skin, a crème or a gel blush is a much better choice than powder. It is more moisturizing, lasts longer, and looks more natural. Crème and gel blushes actually blend into dry skin, whereas powder just sits on top. Remember, when using a crème or gel, to apply it after foundation and before you powder (and if you have dry skin, you will be using very little powder), or it will not go on evenly.

Whenever I wear blush, I feel it's all you see; it never looks natural. What am I doing wrong? How can I make it look more natural?

First, be sure you have chosen the correct shade. If you are using a shade that is too dark or too intense, it will be hard to apply your blush so that it looks natural. Remember to choose a shade that mimics your natural flush (or pinch your cheeks to see the color you need), no darker. You can use a bright, sheer color but never a really dark shade; blush is meant to add color and life to the face, not make it look dark and muddy. Also, be sure you are putting it where it belongs; blush in the wrong place can look unnatural. Lastly, if you have applied your blush and it appears too intense, simply brush loose or pressed facial powder over the color, to mute it and help blend it in.

amy, 30s

Amy's strong jawline is amazing but needs to be slightly softened. The beautiful flush I added to the apples of her cheek was the perfect choice.

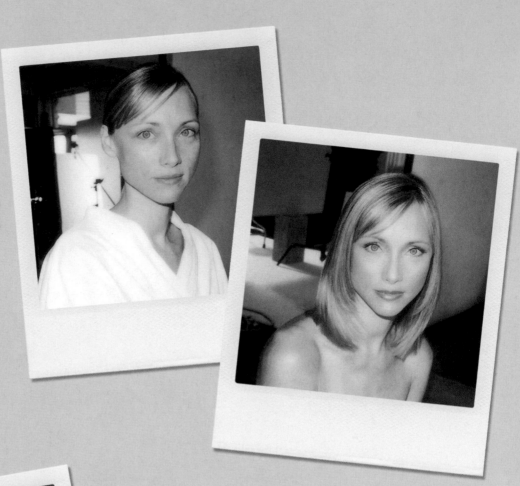

michelle, 20s

I love Michelle's square face, but I wanted to narrow the fullness. Contouring definitely achieved my goal, and an added benefit is the glow it gave her.

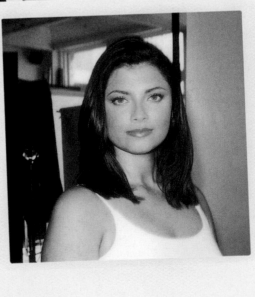

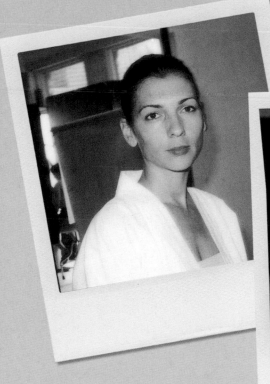

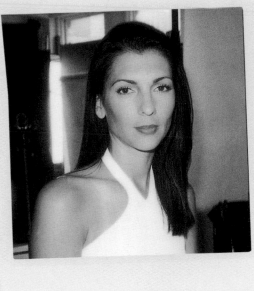

stephanie, 40s

Stephanie has great bone structure, but her face needed color and the definition, to bring out that structure. I love what I was able to accomplish with highlighting and contouring—perfection.

joy, 20s

Now these are lips—perfection. I always say, you know your lips look good if you can look in the mirror and think, I want to kiss myself. Joy had to want to kiss herself.

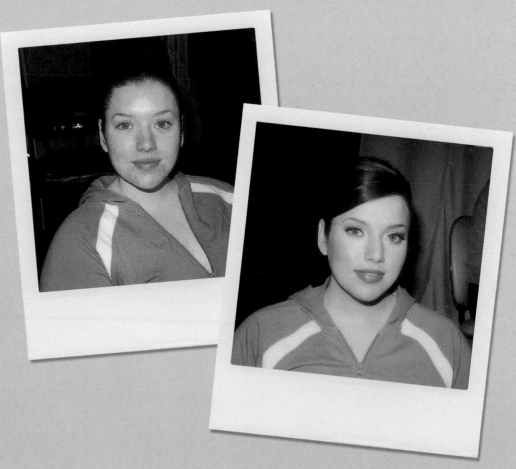

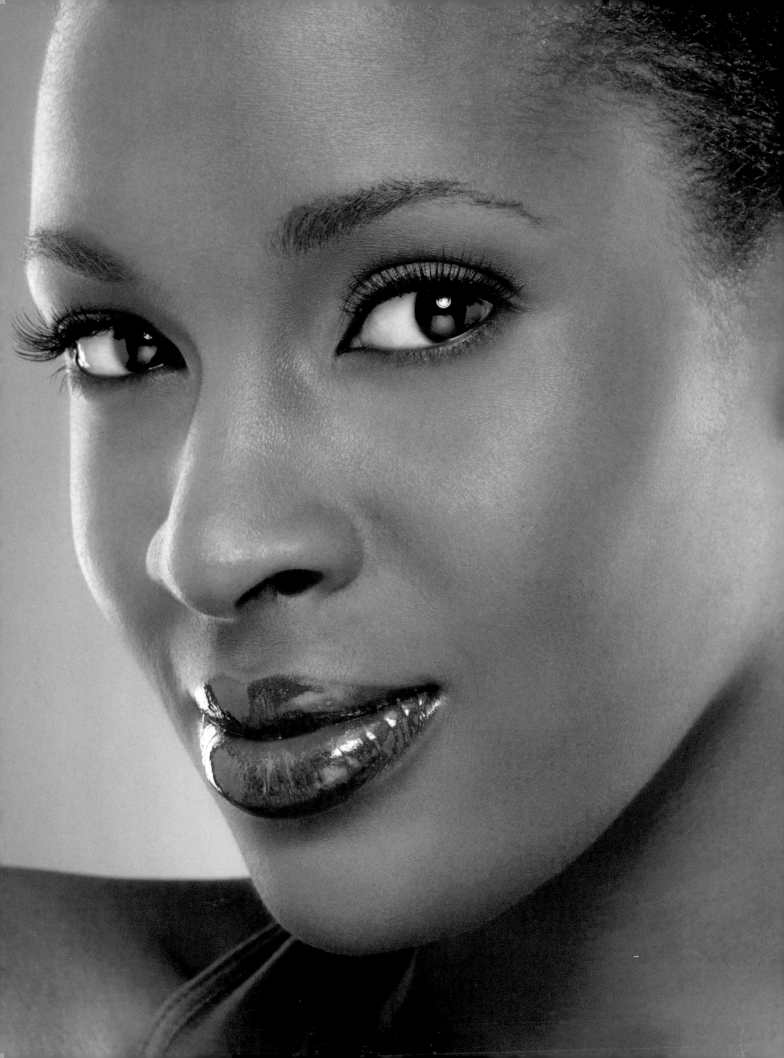

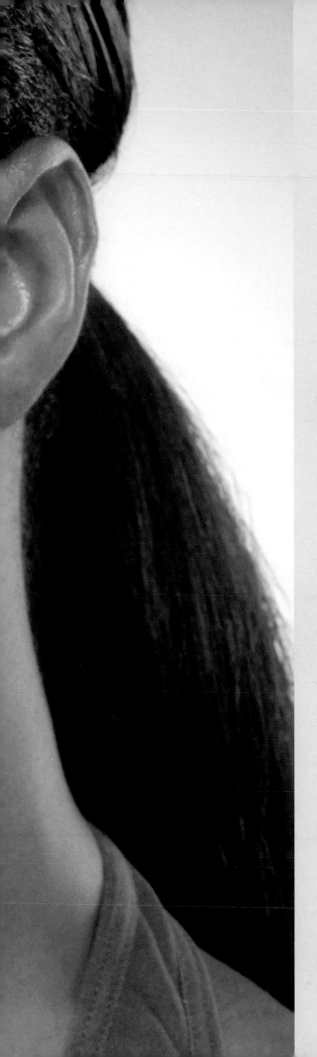

10

lip service

Lip color can do so much for you in your quest for youth. The right shade can make your lips full and youthful, whereas the wrong shade can immediately age you and make your lips look pursed. Lighter shades make your lips look fuller, while darker shades make your lips look thinner. And when it comes to lips, size definitely matters! The size of your lips determines the number of lip color options you have. Fuller lips always make you look younger; unfortunately though, as you age, your lips shrink in size. So our goal is to optimize the size of your lips. (And don't get discouraged—"lighter" does not mean colorless! Your lipstick can be colorful, but a deep shade will minimize the size of your lips.)

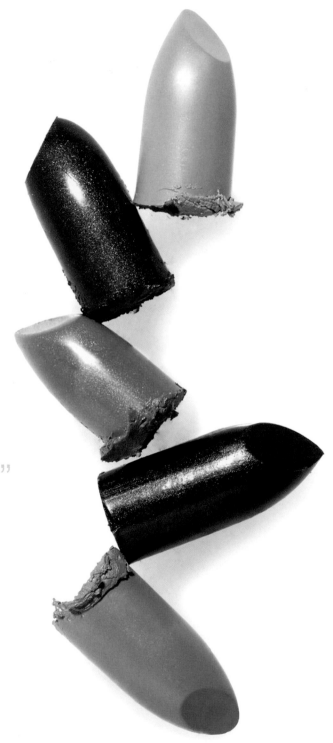

"the fastest way
to look younger
is with a bright,
warm, colorful
shade of lip color"

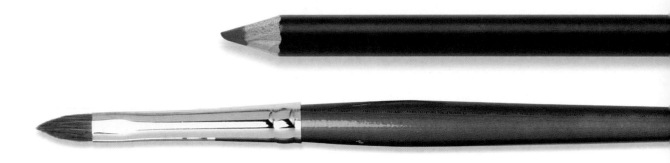

lip a little

If you have ivory/beige skin, the fastest way to age yourself is to wear dark lipstick. (Not so for women with bronze/ebony skin. Because the depth of your skin is deeper, you can pull off a darker shade without looking older.) Even a young girl will look older if she applies a dark shade. So, for a youthful look, go for a brighter, warmer, more colorful shade of lip color. Remember, age strips your face of color; your lips can help you add back some youth. Colorful can equal youthful. A good rule of thumb to avoid aging yourself is to choose a lip color that's no more than two shades darker than your natural lip color.

I am certainly not saying that you cannot wear a rich burgundy or bright red lip color—you can. Just be sure it is the right shade for you. First, be sure your lips are full enough to pull it off. Second, be sure the depth of color will not wash you out (the deeper your skin color, the easier this is to avoid). And last, compensate for the extra depth by adding color to your cheeks and making sure your eyeshadow color choices are softer in depth.

lipstick

If your skin is fair, choose warm pinks and corals or a soft nude color with a peachy undertone. For medium complexions, look for shades with a bit more depth. (Remember, the darker your natural lip color, the darker you can go with your lip color and still look natural and youthful.) For medium skin tones, try a deeper rose or light apricot or a nude color with a rich apricot undertone. Olive-toned skin is most flattered by rich, tawny shades, soft raisins, and a nude with a rich caramel under-tone. Bronze skin definitely benefits from shades with a bit of brown in them. Choose shades such as rich raisin, tawny coffee, or a nude with a dark golden beige undertone. Ebony skin needs richer color choices: a deep walnut, rich plums, and a nude with a dark ginger-toned brown (because your skin color is so deep).

You'll notice that I mentioned nude lip shades for every skin tone. Everyone can wear a soft nude lip color, but by nude, I do not mean colorless. Nude means soft and subtle (kissable). Nude lipstick should never be lighter than your skin. Avoid shades with a white undertone—instead, choose golden, peachy, or pink-tinged hues (for ivory/beige). The perfect nude can be hard to find, so don't be afraid to try on multiple shades, until you find the perfect shade. Always finish with a gloss (glossy nude lips are always more youthful than matte).

Choosing the correct formula for your desired lip look is important. Glossy is always sexy. The shine makes your lips appear fuller and more youthful. If your lips tend to be dry, stay away from matte lipstick. Although the formula wears longer, it can make your lips look and feel even more dehydrated. Crème formulas are always a safe choice, because they tend to work in just about any situation and contain plenty of moisture. Visit page 49 to find the perfect texture for you and your needs.

I know many women think that they can no longer wear lip gloss as they age, but this is completely false. Gloss makes your lips look fuller and more youthful, so it can be your best friend. Just know that all glosses are not the same. Visit page 50 to help you choose the right formula for the results you want.

When choosing the right shade of lip liner, keep one thing in mind: You can *never* go wrong by choosing the same shade as your natural lip color. This shade gives you definition and goes with any lipstick or lip gloss, because it matches your natural lips.

tips:

For the most natural-looking lipstick, choose a shade close to your own lip color, just glossier and slightly deeper.

Putting on lipstick straight from the tube will not blend your lip liner. You should always use a brush to blend your lip liner toward the center of the lips.

To look younger, avoid dark lipstick shades. Paler, brighter colors illuminate and make lips appear fuller, whereas dark colors have a minimizing effect, making lips appear smaller.

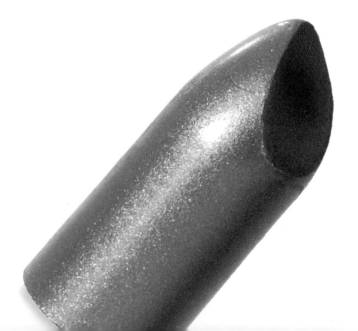

Q&A

I never know which lip liner to choose for what lipstick. Should my lip liner be darker than my lipstick, the same color, or what?

You never want your lip liner to be darker than your lipstick. (If it is, be sure to fill in your entire lip before applying lip color—so you do not look like you ate an Oreo cookie and forgot to wipe your mouth.) A shade the same as your natural lip color always works, because, regardless of the shade you apply on top, your lip liner will match your natural coloring. Keep in mind that your liner color can change your lipstick or gloss shade. For example, if you use a really bright shade of lipstick, it can mute the color of your liner, and using a very deep lipstick shade can lighten the color. So, if you choose a bright lip color and do not want it muted (or softened), choose a lip liner that matches your lipstick or gloss. If you choose a deep lip color and want to avoid having your lip liner lighten the color, choose a shade that matches your lipstick or lip gloss perfectly in depth.

It seems that no matter what shade I choose, my lip color shifts and turns pink. What is happening, and can I prevent it?

If your skin's pH is highly alkaline, the alkalinity in your skin can react with the lipstick pigment and cause it to shift to a pink or orange color. There is no way to stop this from happening, but you can prevent a strong color shift by applying a shade that is the opposite of your shifted color. For instance, if your skin shifts everything to pink, use a shade with a lot of warmth (orange) in it. Instead of becoming super-pink, it will appear neutral. If your lip color tends to shift toward orange, using a shade with a lot of pink in it will help neutralize the orange. One way or the other, if you start out with the complete opposite color, it will not be able to shift all the way to the shade you are trying to avoid. You can use either lip liner or lipstick, or layer the two, to prevent the color shift.

I only wear lip gloss. I know the color won't last as long as lipstick, but is there any way to help it last longer?

Yes, there is a way to get lip gloss to last longer. Before applying your gloss, line and fill in your entire lip with a lip liner that matches your natural lip color. Now, apply a tiny bit of lip balm—the waxier the texture, the better—and apply it over your lip liner. Then apply your gloss. This method helps the color from your gloss last much longer.

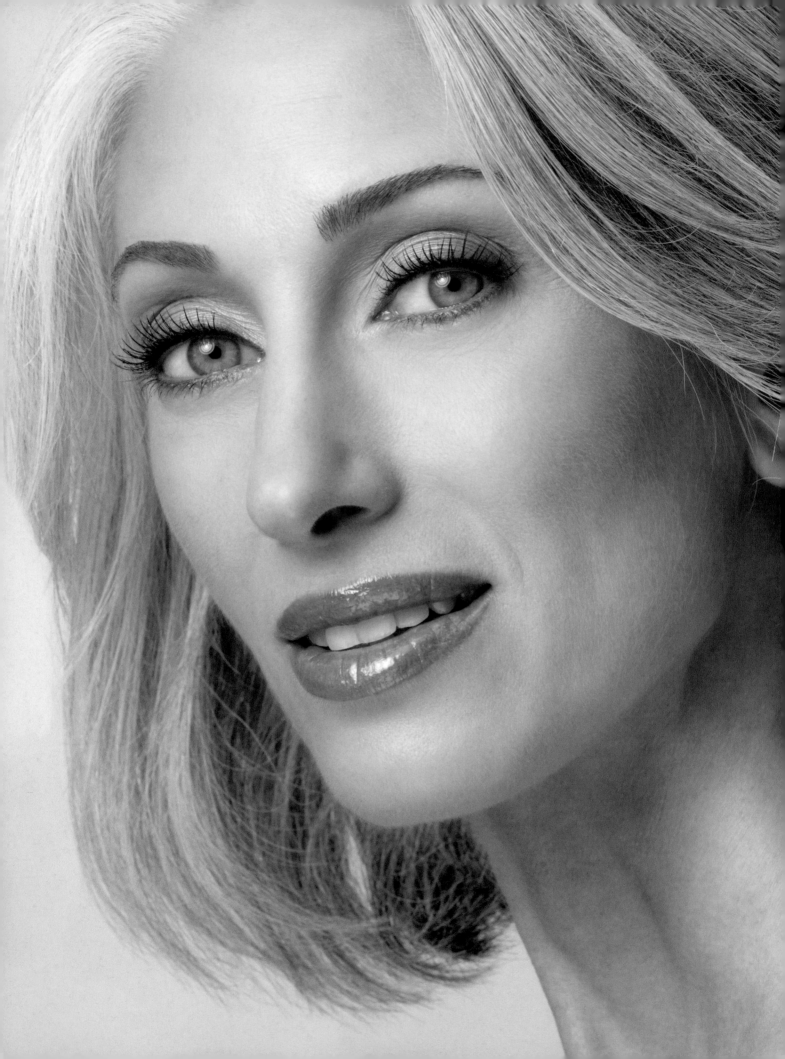

application

To keep your lips looking luscious and youthful, exfoliate them at least once a week. To exfoliate, apply a generous layer of lip balm to your lips, let it soak in for a few minutes, then take a soft baby's toothbrush and brush your lips. (You can also brush them at the same time you brush your teeth.) If you don't have a toothbrush handy, rub them with a nubby-textured washcloth. The balm softens the dry skin so that when you brush (or rub) your lips, you will remove the dry layer of skin, leaving the lips soft and smooth.

I like to use a little lip balm or moisturizer on the lips before I apply lip color, because it helps the lip liner and lipstick go on smoothly and more evenly. Apply the lip balm when you first start applying your makeup, at the same time as your moisturizer. Just before you apply your lip color, blot off the excess. This gives the balm time to soak in. You blot the excess off before applying your lip color, so the balm will not shorten your lip color's wear time.

Lip pencil helps prevent lipstick from feathering and bleeding, but don't stop once you've lined your lips. Be sure to blend the liner inward, so that when your lipstick wears off, you aren't left with just an outline. A lip brush will help give you a more precise application and help your liner and lip color blend better.

Be sure to optimize your entire mouth. Most women don't, tending to draw inside their natural lip line. Most of the time, your lip line actually extends farther than the colored portion of your lip. Use your entire lip! Fuller lips make you look younger, and because you are losing volume in your lips, you definitely want to optimize what you do have.

To apply your lip liner to the top lip, begin with a V in the "cupid's bow," or center curve of the lips. Bring the liner up and around the curves of your bow. Then, starting at the outer corners, draw small, feathery strokes to meet the center bow. Don't worry if the line is not consistent—you can use a lip brush to blend the line and make it look more natural.

For the lower lip, first accentuate the lower curve of the lip, then make small feather-like strokes from the outer corners, moving towards the center. Remember to use your entire lip: Take the color to the almost invisible line just at the edge of the colored part of your lips. Finally, blend with a lip brush to make the liner look its most natural.

Your lips are now ready for you to apply your lipstick and gloss.

You can use a brush, your fingers, or a tube to apply your lipstick, but if it's applied with a brush, it will usually last longer and look much more precise. For more intense color, apply it straight from the tube, but it will be harder to cover the smaller, detailed areas of the lips. If you do apply lip color straight from the tube, go back over it with a brush for a better blend.

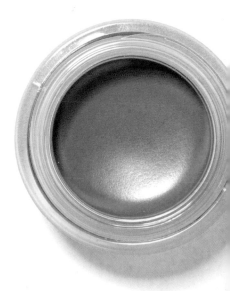

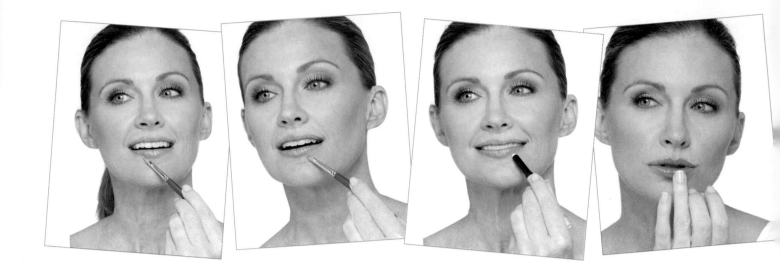

 Q&A

Regardless of whether I wear lipstick or lip gloss, my lip color bleeds. Is there any way to prevent this?

You have multiple options to prevent bleeding, but your goal is always the same: You want to create a dam (or ledge), so nothing can bleed outward. Filling in the fine lines around your mouth will also help to prevent bleeding. Here are some products and techniques to consider:

1. Use lip liner: this is your first line of defense to prevent bleeding.

2. Dip a cotton swab into loose powder and run it along the outer edge of your lip.

3. Dab some concealer onto your concealer brush and apply it around the mouth, just at the edge of the lip line. This creates a dam, so nothing can bleed outward, and also fills in any fine lines. This is one of the most effective ways to prevent bleeding without buying additional products.

4. You can purchase products designed to create a dam (or ledge) for you. They have a waxy, velvety texture. The great thing is that they are clear, so they never show. To use them, apply the product around the outer edge of your lip. This is the absolute best way to prevent bleeding.

5. Lastly, if you want to skip the extra steps and extra product, you can simply apply less lipstick, so that it will not slide and bleed. Do what I call staining your lips: Instead of applying your lipstick with a brush or from the tube (this puts a lot more product on your lips), dab it on with your fingers. This creates a stain on your lips, rather than a full layer of lipstick.

tips:

Color adheres better to a smooth surface, so exfoliate your lips at least once a week.

Your lip liner should never be visible after you have applied your lipstick and/or gloss.

Do I have to wear lip liner?

There is no rule stating that you have to wear lip liner, but it does three things for you, and I find most women want at least one of these three things to happen:

1. Lip liner can help define your mouth and reshape your lips if they are uneven, giving your lips a nice edge.
2. Lip liner can help prevent your lip color from bleeding.
3. Lip liner can help your lipstick last longer, especially if you fill in your lips with liner before applying your lip color. I always fill in at least halfway toward the center of the mouth with lip liner before I apply lipstick.

Do you recommend all-day lip color products?

Never expect lipstick to last all day. I know there are formulas that claim all-day wear, but I personally do not think you should ever want anything on your lips for that length of time (except maybe someone else's lips). Formulas that last all day make the lips look parched and dry. These products contain stains that (unless your lips are freshly exfoliated) adhere unevenly to the dry areas of your lips, causing your lipstick to appear splotchy and dehydrated. But worst of all, these formulas will make your lips look old, instead of youthful.

It seems my lip color never lasts, how can I get longer wear out of my lip color?

There are many ways to get your lip color to last. I have tried them all and have found in the end there is one way that really works best and keeps your lips feeling their most supple.

1. Conceal the entire lip area with concealer or foundation—include your natural lip line as well

tips:

To make sure your lip liner provides the most natural application, warm it between your fingers for a couple of seconds before applying it.

Applying your lip gloss with a brush will make it appear shinier than if you apply it with a sponge tip.

To keep lipstick from smearing onto your teeth, stick your finger in your mouth after application, purse your lips around it, and pull it out. This removes any color on the inside of your lips and keeps it from smearing onto your teeth.

as your lip. This hides any discoloration just outside your lip line and creates a better edge. It also creates a blank canvas on which to apply your lip color.

2. Use lip liner to line the outer edges of your lips and then fill in the entire lip area (use the side of the pencil, rather than the point, for a more even application of color). This is the first line of defense in getting your lip color to last. Lip liner has a drier texture than lipstick, so it lasts longer.

3. Next, apply your lipstick, then gently blot your lips with a tissue. Blotting removes the moisture from this layer, yet leaves a deposit of lipstick pigment. Reapply your lipstick, but, this time, do not blot. Layering color like this provides double the pigment deposit, which increases wear time.

4. Finish with a dot of lip gloss in the center of the lips, to attract light and make your lips look fuller and more youthful.

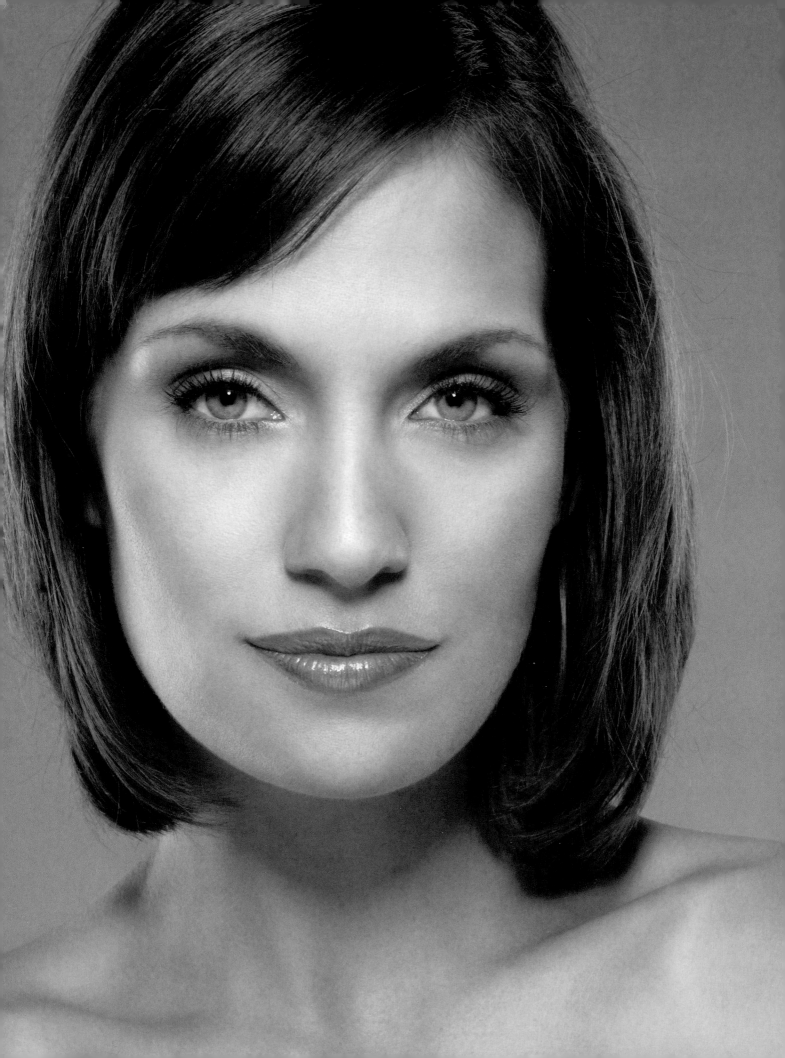

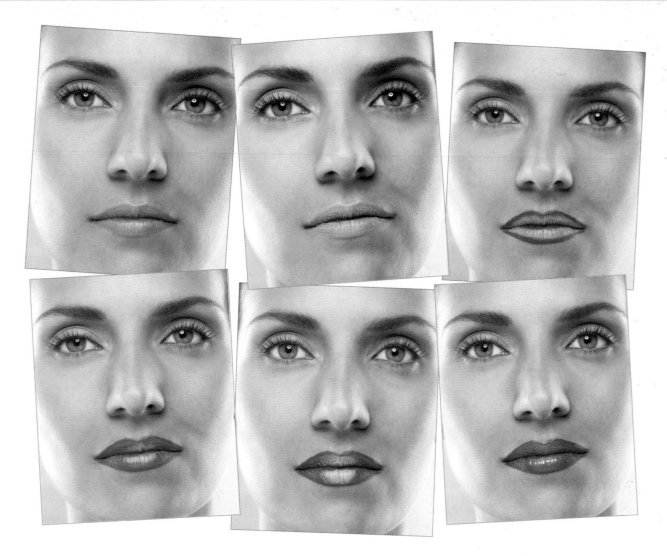

fuller lips

I'm sure you already know that fuller lips make you look younger, because lips lose fullness as they age. Perhaps your lips are not as full as you would like them to be, but you don't want to resort to injections. Try this *looking younger* trade secret. It's a way to apply your lip color that makes your lips look fuller but completely natural and, of course, younger.

1. Erase your existing lip line with concealer or foundation. This creates a fresh canvas onto which you can create a whole new lip line.

2. Using a natural-toned lip pencil (not dark, but neutral and natural), draw a line just slightly above your natural lip across the top and slightly below your lip along your bottom lip line. Don't exaggerate the line—just draw it slightly above your top and slightly below your bottom lip line.

3. Now, fill in your lips with the lip liner, except for the very center of your top and bottom lips.

4. Next, dab a little concealer in the center of your top and bottom lip and then apply your lipstick. The lipstick will mix with the concealer and leave the center of your lips lighter, making them appear fuller.

5. To finish, apply a light, shimmery lip gloss to the center of your lips, over your lipstick (blending it outward). The gloss reflects light and helps your lips appear even fuller.

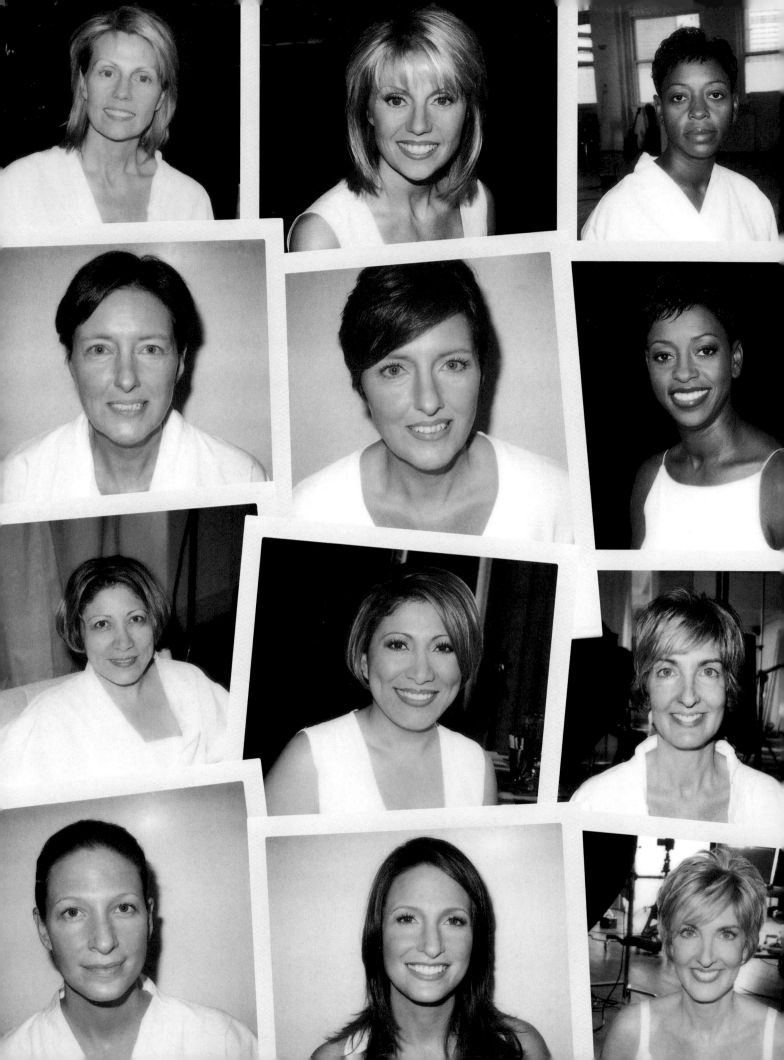

"there is no such thing as an unattractive woman—just a woman who has not discovered the benefits of makeup"

part three | being beautiful now and at every age

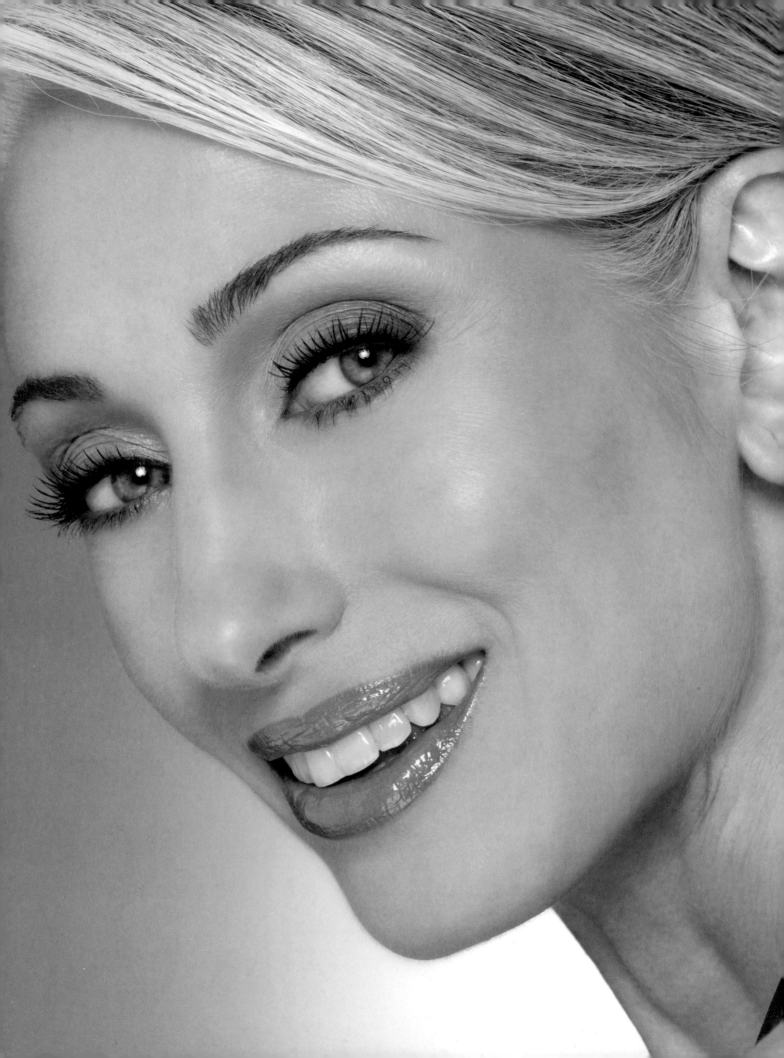

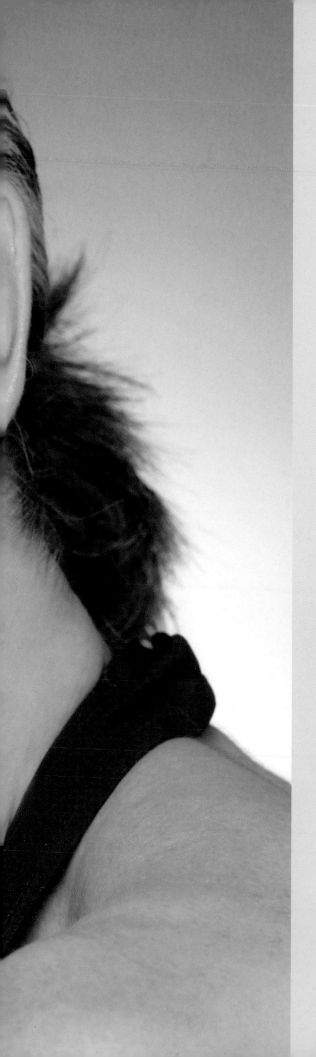

11

becoming younger, step by step

Nothing demonstrates the transformation that can take place when you make the right makeup choices better than a step-by-step tutorial. In this chapter, you will see just how easy and effective the process of making yourself look your most youthful really is. And I think you'll enjoy watching the journey to looking younger take place, one step at a time. I know I always do!

First, however, I'd like to give you a quick review of the application process, so it will be easy for you, too, to become younger, step by step. Women often ask me if there's a "right" order to apply makeup. The order in which you put on your makeup varies, depending on what works best for you—there are no set rules. Following is the order of application that I like to use. But don't think you have to copy it; feel free to do what works best for you.

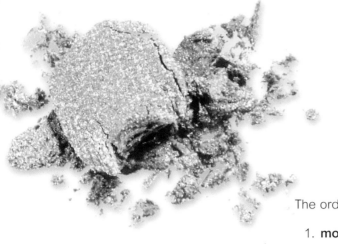

The order I recommend and use is this:

1. **moisturizer** (not up for debate, this *must* go first)
2. **sunscreen** (unless your moisturizer already contains it)
3. **eye crème** (again, a must)
4. **lip balm**
5. **primer**
6. **concealer**
7. **foundation**
8. **powder**
9. **brows**
10. **eyeshadow**
11. **eyeliner**
12. **lashes**
13. **bronzer**
14. **blush**
15. **lip liner**
16. **lipstick**
17. **lip gloss**

As I show Susan's transformation and go through each application in the pages that follow, I'll tell you when something *must* be applied in a certain order. I will share with you what I find works best for my clients, and I'll tell you why I like my order better than others. Some of my reasons may make sense to you, and some may not. For now, just enjoy the transformation. You will find that, in the end, my simple techniques have achieved our goal: a more youthful, radiant beauty. I suggest that you use this order as a starting point. As you work with the steps on your own and discover what works best for you, feel free to create an order that works for you.

susan's transformation

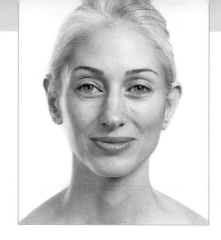

Susan begins by prepping her face. First she applies moisturizer, choosing the right formula for her skin type. Susan makes sure to let her moisturizer dry completely (this is paramount—it ensures that everything applied after goes on evenly). Next, she applies sunscreen and allows it to dry and absorb into her skin. Now, she applies a healthy dose of eye crème, which will keep the area under the eye looking smooth and supple while helping her make-up go on more evenly. She then applies a face primer, to help her makeup last all day and prevent it from settling into fine lines. Finally, she applies a generous dose of lip balm. Susan has basically prepared her canvas and is now ready for color.

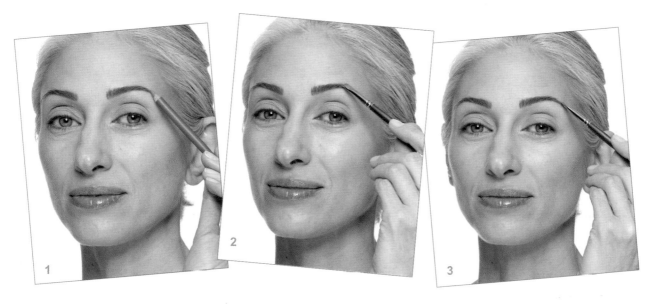

Susan has applied concealer to any and all imperfections, finishing by applying a layer to her eyelids (giving her the perfect blank canvas for all eyeshadow color that will be applied later). It's now time for her to apply foundation, the next step in creating the illusion of flawless, youthful-looking skin. Susan has already shaped her eyebrows to perfection, using the steps outlined on page 76. Now she wants to fine-tune and add some definition to her brows, so they are the perfect frame for her beautiful blue eyes.

She starts shaping by using a pencil to fill in sparse areas (1) and create the perfect brow shape (remember, fuller brows look younger). She follows this step by tracing her pencil strokes exactly with a stiff, short-bristled, angled brush (2). The brush helps to blend the pencil and make it look more natural.

After this, Susan follows the same steps again, but this time, she dips the brush in a bit of brow powder to set the pencil (3). She finishes by going back over everything with a full (toothbrush-shaped) brow brush, brushing the brow hairs upward and into place and resulting in the ultimate blend and natural finish. (Remember, if you have unruly brow hair, now is the time to use brow gel, to keep everything under control throughout the day.)

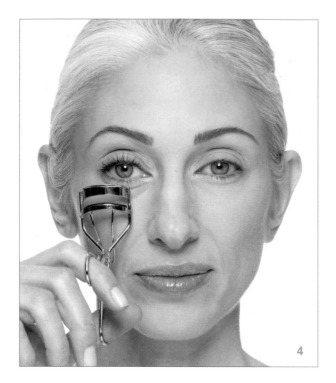

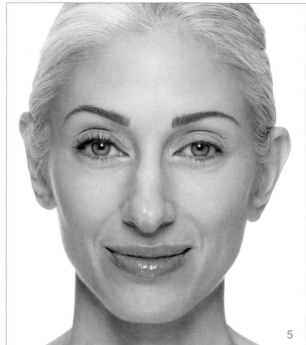

Time for one of my favorite tricks in the whole application process: curling the lashes. Starting with clean lashes, Susan crimp-curls her eyelashes. You can see from the picture (4), with one curled and the other not, what a difference curling makes! The eye with curled lashes looks younger, bigger, and more open (5). This is a must. At this point, Susan applies her first layer of mascara to her upper lashes.

Using one of her favorite highlight eyeshadow colors, Susan applies shadow to her lid and brow bone. She follows it by applying her midtone color, starting from the outside corner of the crease and brushing it across the lid, in the crease, all the way into the inside corner of the lid (6). She also applies the midtone shade all along her lower lash line, starting from the outside corner and working across to the inside corner. Using the midtone color here first will help blend everything she applies to this area later.

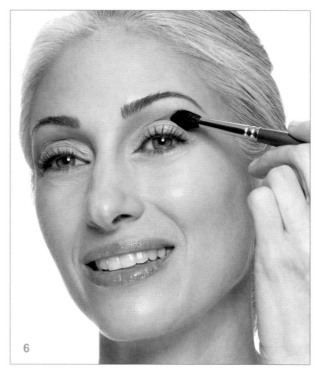

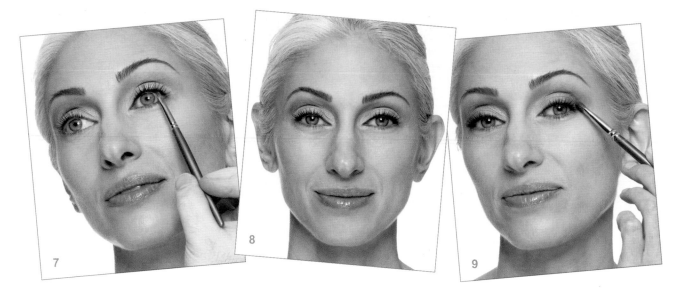

Now it's time for my secret to perfect eye definition. First, Susan dips a narrow, flat, short-bristle brush into black eyeshadow. She then pushes the brush up into the lash line, right at the base of her lashes (at the root, where they grow out of the lid, not on the wet tissue of the lid), depositing the color. She starts from the outside corner and works all the way across to the inside corner, so the definition extends all the way across her lid (7). This helps define the eye without making it look heavily lined, while giving the lashes the illusion of appearing much thicker (8).

The next step is applying the contour color. Starting from the outside corner of the upper lid, Susan brushes color all the way across the upper lash line and up into the outer corner of the crease (9), about a third of the way across the crease. She follows by using a clean, fluffy blending brush to brush across the entire lid and create a perfect blend. Next, Susan uses a wide, flat eyeliner brush with a high concentration of contour shadow to create a definite line along her upper lash line. This technique gives definition, like eyeliner does, but looks softer and less harsh. Susan then applies the second layer of mascara to her upper lashes.

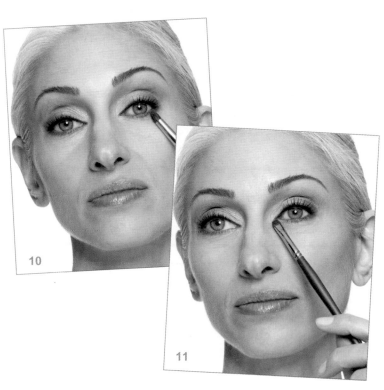

Susan applies her contour color (using the right brush), starting from the outside corner and moving across to the inside corner of her lower lash line (10). This application technique gives her the perfect definition, while looking subtle. I prefer a very soft definition like this along the lower lash line.

To open up the eye and create a youthful, wide-eyed effect, Susan applies her highlight shade right at the inside corner of her lower lash line (11). Next, she applies her third and final layer of mascara to the upper lashes. Spacing out the mascara applications gives Susan's top lashes plenty of time to dry between layers, and because they are thin layers, there's no clumping. She then applies a thin coat of mascara to her lower lashes (only one coat here for softness and subtle definition).

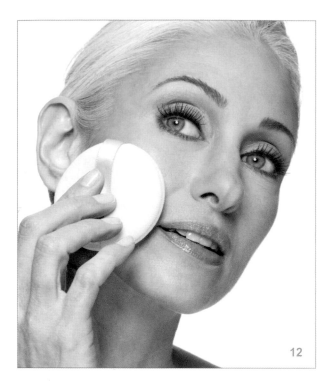

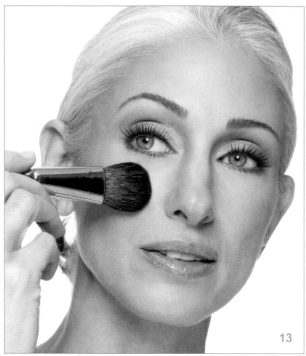

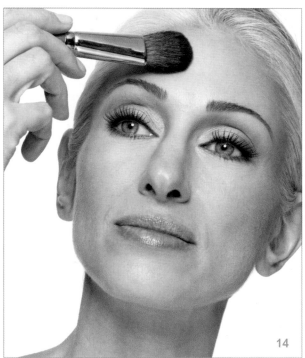

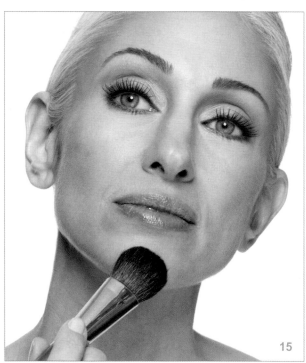

Susan sets her makeup with powder to make sure it lasts all day. It will also make her blush and bronzer go on and blend better. Susan concentrates her powder on the areas that become shiny the fastest. (You do not have to powder your entire face if your skin tends to be dry, but be sure to powder the areas that need setting.) Susan uses a powder puff for more powder coverage and smooth application, pushing the powder into the skin and helping it to become one with her skin (12), then uses a brush to remove the excess (13–15). For a lighter application, she can use a brush to dust the powder over the areas that need oil absorption and setting.

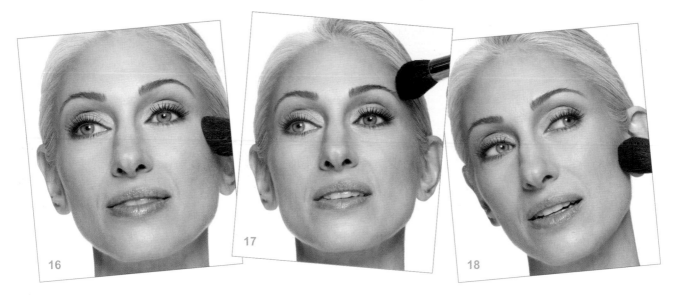

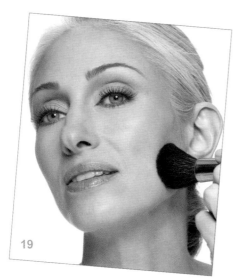

Now for the youthful glow. Susan applies the perfect shade of matte bronzer to give her skin a beautiful kiss of color. She starts at the back of her cheekbone and sweeps it toward the apple of her cheek and back (16). She then blends the bronzer up onto her temples (17) and down toward her jawline (18–19), giving her skin a beautiful wash of color.

For a flush of youthful color, Susan uses a full, soft, tapered brush and a fresh, sheer, bright blush and applies it back toward her bronzed cheekbones to "pop" the apples of her cheeks (20). The sheer, bright color made Susan look much younger than she would have had she used a dark, intense shade, which would have been too harsh.

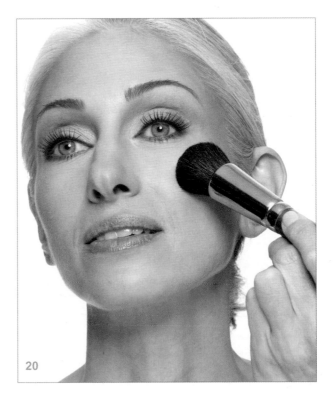

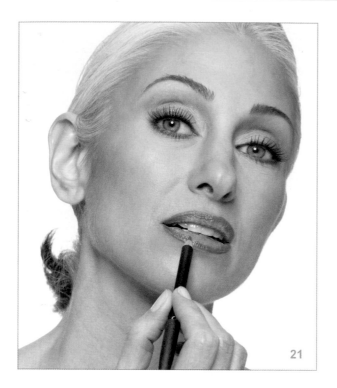

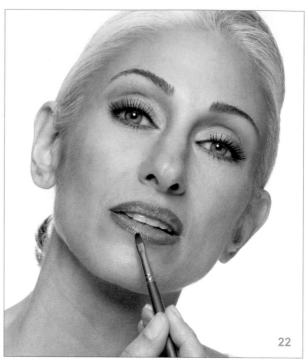

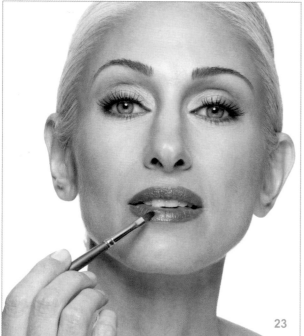

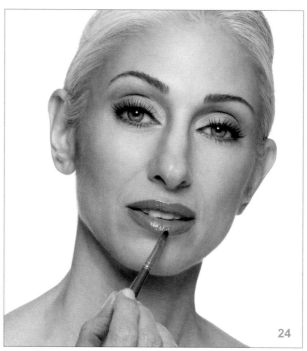

Susan lines her lips with a natural tone of lip liner, just a couple of shades deeper than her natural lip color. She does not stop with a line around her lips; instead, she brings the color toward the center of her lips (21), which helps her lip color stay on and her lip liner blend better. She then uses her lip brush to blend the liner even more, for the most natural effect (22).

With a lip brush, Susan applies the perfect shade of lipstick—natural, but bright enough to add color to her face, with a hint of coral to it (23). She follows it by applying a great lip gloss (24).

Susan's transformation is truly proof that the right color choices and the right placement of color can bring you to the end result of youthful beauty. Remember, play and experiment with color to create the most beautiful you!

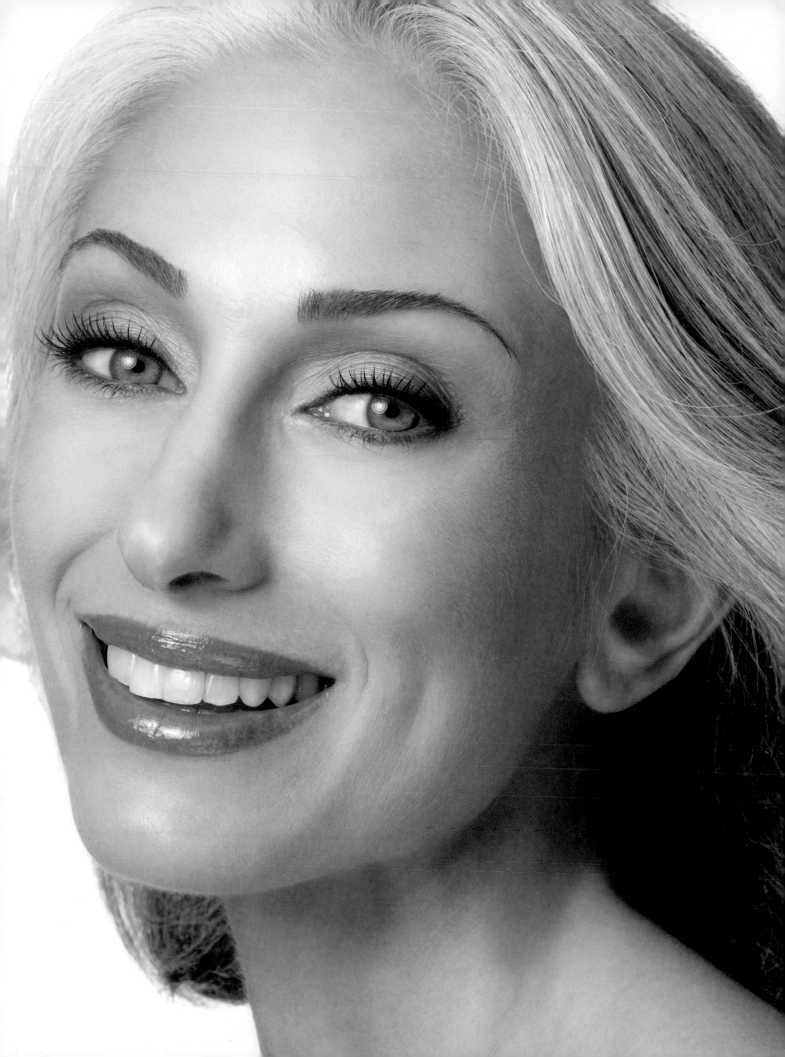

12

looking younger
transformations

So far, you've seen a lot of specific ways to bring out your beauty, from choosing the right foundation to shaping your brows to making your lips look full and luscious. In the previous chapter, you saw how to put all my looking younger secrets together to bring out your inner beauty. But what if you're not convinced that you can actually do it yourself? You may be thinking, "I don't look like Susan in Chapter 11. Will Robert's techniques really work for me?"

The answer is yes, absolutely. Over the years, I've watched thousands of women bring out their true beauty using my techniques. But I'm also a big believer in the school of thought that seeing is believing. So in this chapter, I'm going to show you dozens of real-life transformations. You'll be able to see these wonderful effects on women of all ages, races, skin types, and face shapes. I can guarantee that, once you've paged through this chapter, you'll be a believer, too!

Take a look at all the before-and-afters, and zero in on the women who look most like you. Check out the products and techniques I used to bring out their true beauty, and you'll have a great starting point for your own transformation. What are you waiting for?

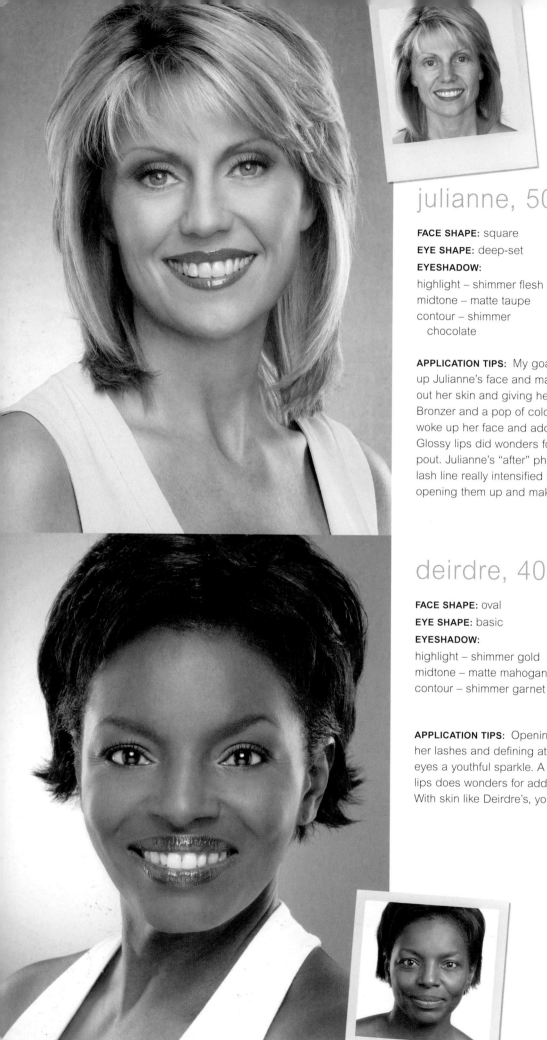

julianne, 50s

FACE SHAPE: square
EYE SHAPE: deep-set
EYESHADOW:
highlight – shimmer flesh
midtone – matte taupe
contour – shimmer
   chocolate

EYELINER: dark brown
BLUSH: soft peach
LIP LINER: flesh
LIPSTICK: creamy toffee
LIP GLOSS: creamy nude

APPLICATION TIPS: My goal of course was to brighten up Julianne's face and make her look younger. Evening out her skin and giving her a warm glow took years off. Bronzer and a pop of color on the apples of her cheeks woke up her face and added the color she needed. Glossy lips did wonders for giving her a sexy, youthful pout. Julianne's "after" photo shows how defining at the lash line really intensified the blue in her eyes, as well as opening them up and making them look younger.

deirdre, 40s

FACE SHAPE: oval
EYE SHAPE: basic
EYESHADOW:
highlight – shimmer gold
midtone – matte mahogany
contour – shimmer garnet

EYELINER: black
BLUSH: soft brick
LIP LINER: mahogany
LIPSTICK: rich raisin
LIP GLOSS: shimmer bronze

APPLICATION TIPS: Opening up Deirdre's eyes by curling her lashes and defining at her lash line really gives her eyes a youthful sparkle. A nice, soft shot of color on her lips does wonders for adding color and life to her face. With skin like Deirdre's, you can't help but look young!

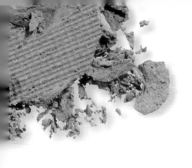

eleanor, 30s

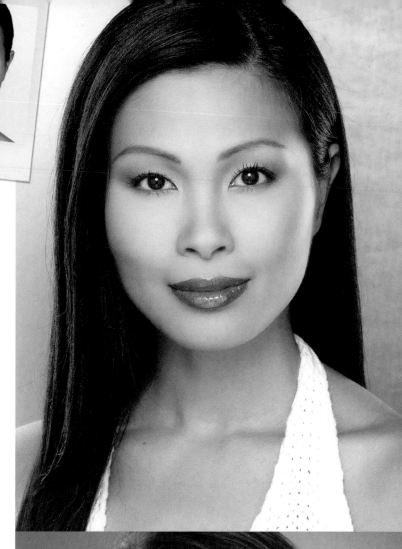

FACE SHAPE: round
EYE SHAPE: hooded
EYESHADOW:
highlight – shimmer flesh
midtone – matte dark taupe
contour – shimmer
   chocolate

EYELINER: dark brown
BLUSH: soft apricot
LIP LINER: caramel
LIPSTICK: creamy toffee
LIP GLOSS: shimmer rose

APPLICATION TIPS: With Eleanor, my biggest goal was to really define her eyes and open them up. By applying eyeshadow for her specific eye shape and choosing the right shades, I achieved my goal. A beautiful warm glow and glossy, sexy lips certainly didn't hurt, either!

kim, 30s

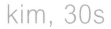

FACE SHAPE: square
EYE SHAPE: basic
EYESHADOW:
highlight – shimmer flesh
midtone – matte taupe
contour – shimmer
   chocolate

EYELINER: bronze
BLUSH: soft peach
LIP LINER: flesh
LIPSTICK: peachy nude
LIP GLOSS: shimmer
   peachy nude

APPLICATION TIPS: One of the most effective techniques for Kim was giving her fuller brows. Note how well they frame her eyes and give them the attention they need. Remember, fuller brows always make you look younger. Kim's age (only thirty) didn't hurt, but you can see that, even for her, the right color choices and application techniques help her look her most youthful and beautiful.

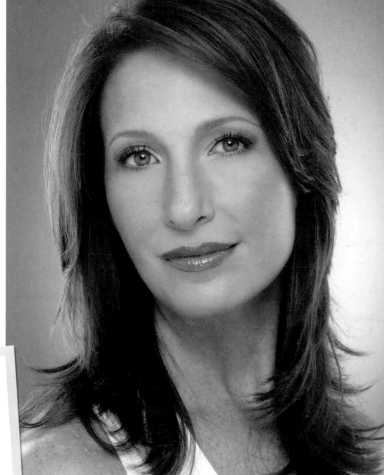

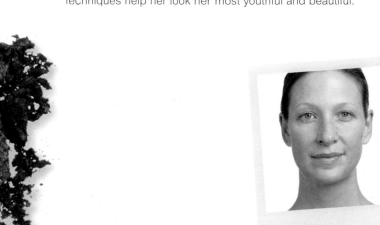

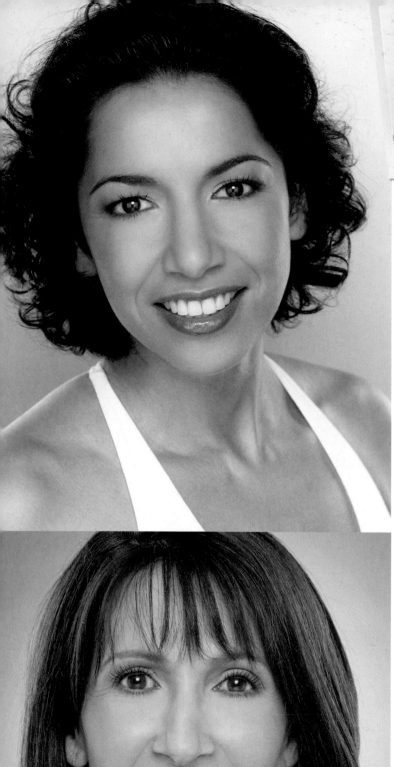

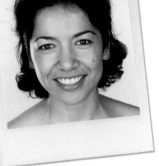

lydia, 40s

FACE SHAPE: pear
EYE SHAPE: hooded
EYESHADOW:
highlight – shimmer flesh
midtone – matte caramel
contour – shimmer garnet

EYELINER: dark brown
BLUSH: soft apricot
LIP LINER: caramel
LIPSTICK: peachy nude
LIP GLOSS: shimmer rose

APPLICATION TIPS: Lydia's biggest problem is her heavy, hooded eyelids. Visually pushing back her eyelids with the right eyeshadow application immediately wakes up her face and makes her look younger. Warming up her skin and giving her an amazing glow was a big help, as well.

rita, 50s

FACE SHAPE: oval
EYE SHAPE: basic
EYESHADOW:
highlight – matte nude/
   shimmer flesh
midtone – matte taupe
contour – matte brown

EYELINER: bronze
BLUSH: soft peach
LIP LINER: flesh
LIPSTICK: soft peach
LIP GLOSS: creamy nude

APPLICATION TIPS: For Rita, my goal was to liven up her face and draw attention to her best feature: her eyes. Without the right eye makeup, you can't really see her eyes, but after her makeover, with the right shade choices and application, they stand out and really look youthful. Giving her a beautiful, even complexion (hiding the little things we did not want to see) also really helps put focus on her eyes.

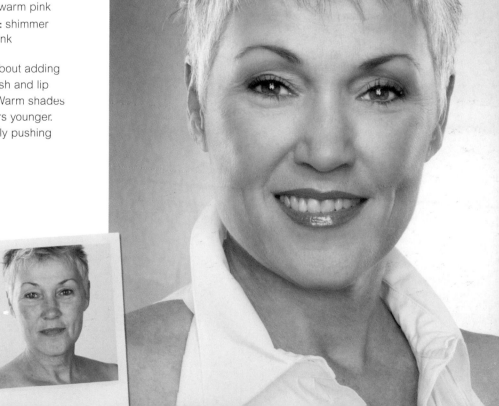

joyce, 70s

FACE SHAPE: pear
EYE SHAPE: hooded
EYESHADOW:

highlight – matte nude
midtone – matte taupe
contour – matte brown

EYELINER: bronze
BLUSH: soft peach
LIP LINER: fleshy pink
LIPSTICK: coral
LIP GLOSS: shimmer peach

APPLICATION TIPS: Adding color and definition took years off Joyce's appearance. Many women Joyce's age think they should just give up. Never! By defining her features but choosing softer colors, I gave her the look of youth she deserved. Beautiful, even skin really helped, as well. Most important is a young spirit, which she obviously has. If every woman looked as good as Joyce does at her age, we would all be in trouble!

wanda, 50s

FACE SHAPE: oval
EYE SHAPE: hooded
EYESHADOW:

highlight – matte nude
midtone – matte dark taupe
contour – matte brown

EYELINER: dark brown
BLUSH: warm pink
LIP LINER: fleshy pink
LIPSTICK: warm pink
LIP GLOSS: shimmer
warm pink

APPLICATION TIPS: For Wanda, it was all about adding color and life to her face, so I chose a blush and lip colors that really added warmth and life. Warm shades (even warm pinks) will make you look years younger. Defining Wanda's eyes helped, too. Visually pushing back her hooded lids did the trick.

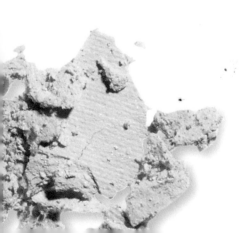

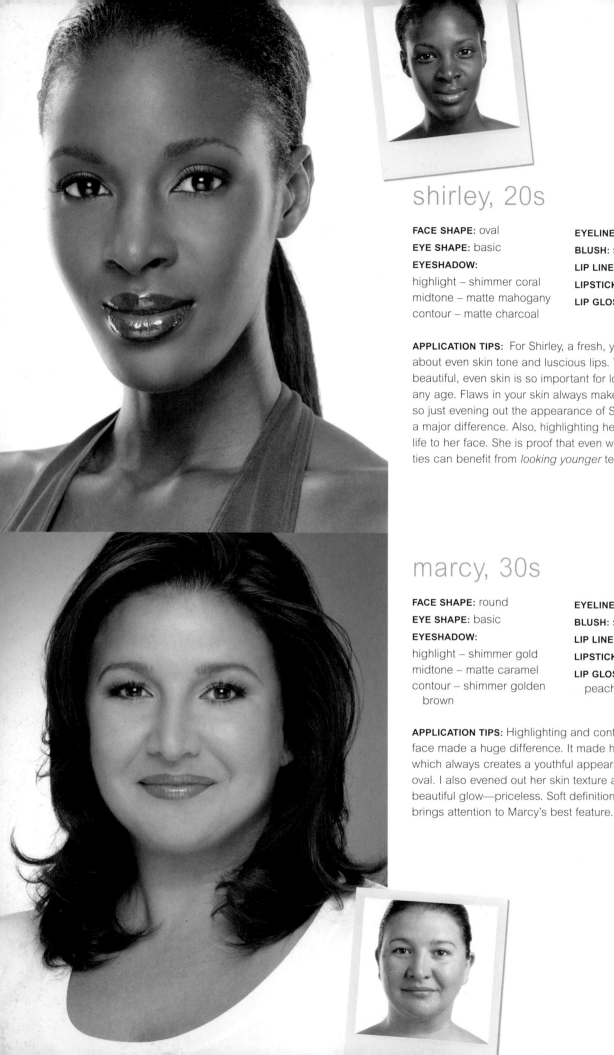

shirley, 20s

FACE SHAPE: oval
EYE SHAPE: basic
EYESHADOW:
highlight – shimmer coral
midtone – matte mahogany
contour – matte charcoal

EYELINER: black
BLUSH: soft brick
LIP LINER: mahogany
LIPSTICK: rich raisin
LIP GLOSS: shimmer berry

APPLICATION TIPS: For Shirley, a fresh, youthful look was all about even skin tone and luscious lips. The appearance of beautiful, even skin is so important for looking younger at any age. Flaws in your skin always make you look older, so just evening out the appearance of Shirley's skin made a major difference. Also, highlighting her skin really added life to her face. She is proof that even women in their twenties can benefit from *looking younger* techniques.

marcy, 30s

FACE SHAPE: round
EYE SHAPE: basic
EYESHADOW:
highlight – shimmer gold
midtone – matte caramel
contour – shimmer golden
   brown

EYELINER: dark brown
BLUSH: soft apricot
LIP LINER: flesh
LIPSTICK: creamy toffee
LIP GLOSS: shimmer
   peachy nude

APPLICATION TIPS: Highlighting and contouring Marcy's face made a huge difference. It made her face look softer, which always creates a youthful appearance, and more oval. I also evened out her skin texture and gave her a beautiful glow—priceless. Soft definition for her eyes really brings attention to Marcy's best feature.

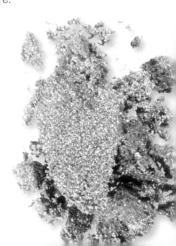

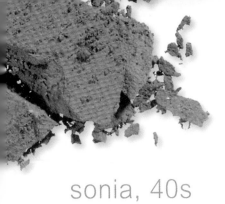

sonia, 40s

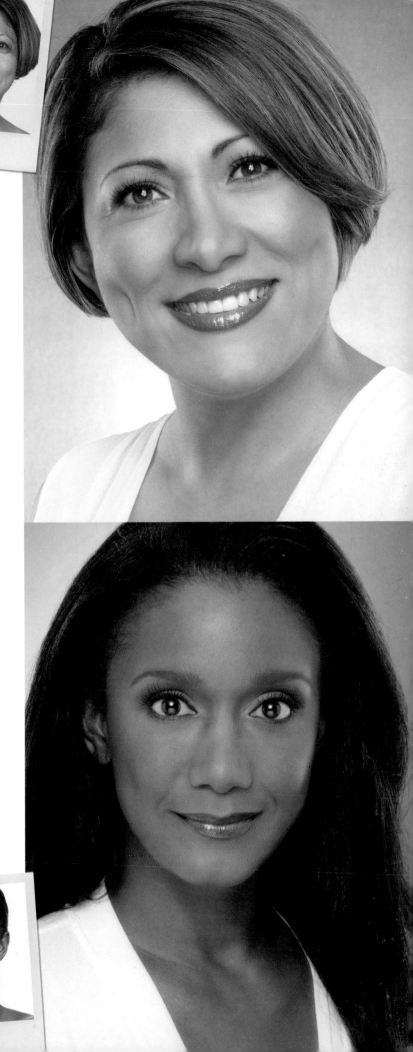

FACE SHAPE: pear
EYE SHAPE: hooded
EYESHADOW:
highlight – shimmer gold
midtone – matte caramel
contour – shimmer golden
    brown

EYELINER: dark brown
BLUSH: soft apricot
LIP LINER: caramel
LIPSTICK: creamy toffee
LIP GLOSS: shimmer
    peachy nude

APPLICATION TIPS: For Sonia, looking younger was all about adding color and opening up her eyes. You can see how she benefited from defining her eyes and visually pushing back her eyelid with eyeshadow. It really made her eyes appear larger. Adding needed color and glow to her cheeks and skin did wonders, too.

alex, 40s

FACE SHAPE: square
EYE SHAPE: basic
EYESHADOW:
highlight – shimmer gold
midtone – matte ginger
contour – matte charcoal

EYELINER: black
BLUSH: soft brick
LIP LINER: mahogany
LIPSTICK: rich raisin
LIP GLOSS: shimmer
    bronze

APPLICATION TIPS: Nothing beats beautiful, even, glowing skin, and that made all the difference for Alex. Making her face look more oval by highlighting the high points and adding a soft glow of color to the cheeks makes her look much more youthful. A glossy, luscious, sexy smile is not hurting her, either. You just know from that spark in her eyes that there is some danger ahead.

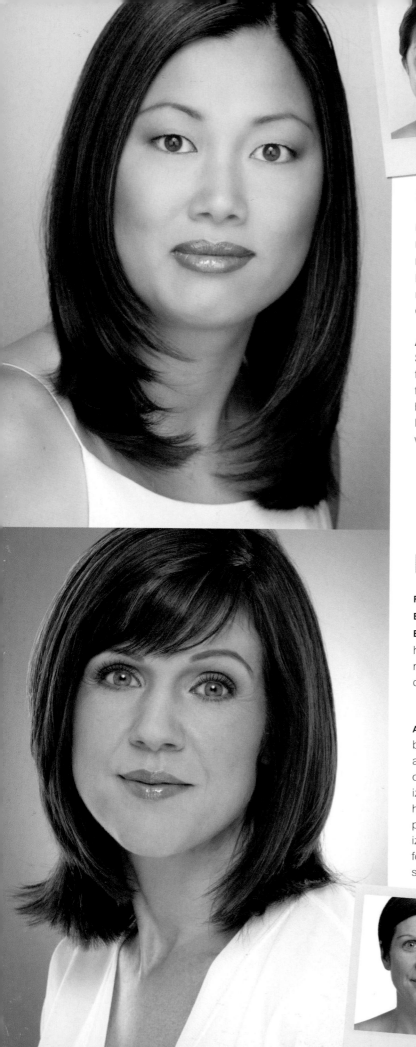

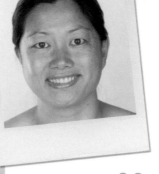

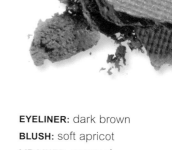

susan, 30s

FACE SHAPE: round
EYE SHAPE: hooded
EYESHADOW:

highlight – shimmer flesh
midtone – matte dark taupe
contour – matte brown

EYELINER: dark brown
BLUSH: soft apricot
LIP LINER: caramel
LIPSTICK: creamy toffee
LIP GLOSS: shimmer peach

APPLICATION TIPS: Beautiful skin and gorgeous lips are all Susan needed to look younger. Making sure that her skin tone was even and that you could not see discoloration took years off her age. I also added a beautiful glow to her cheeks and contouring to her face. With lips like that, I just had to make them full and sexy. How could we live without lip gloss?

kathy, 40s

FACE SHAPE: square
EYE SHAPE: deep-set
EYESHADOW:

highlight – shimmer beige
midtone – matte taupe
contour – shimmer
    chocolate

EYELINER: rich brown
BLUSH: apricot
LIP LINER: warm caramel
LIPSTICK: soft peach
LIP GLOSS: shimmer coral

APPLICATION TIPS: Kathy is the perfect example of how fuller brows can make you look younger. I layered brow pencil and eyebrow powder to fill in and create youthful brows to disguise the originals that she had over-tweezed. Moisturizing extra well and evening out her skin really minimized her fine lines and gave her skin a supple glow. Of course, prepping your skin before makeup is a must! After moisturizing Kathy's skin, I used a foundation primer to help prevent foundation and powder from settling into her fine lines, a step I recommend to anyone who wants to look younger.

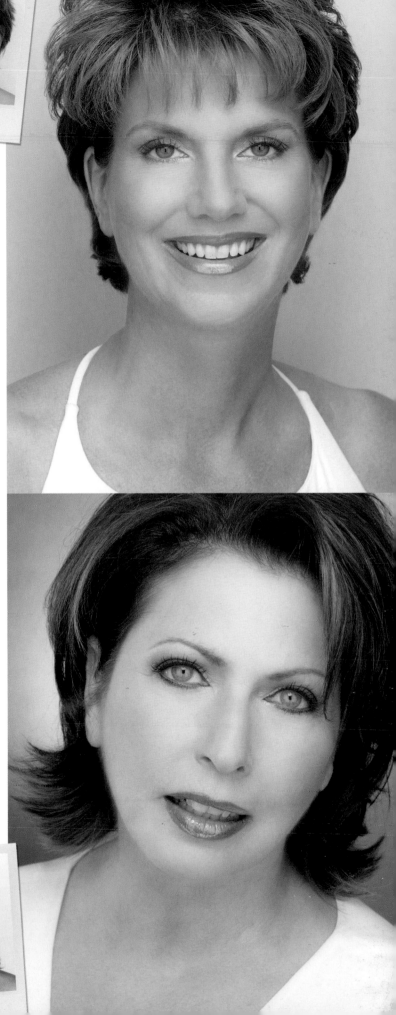

linda, 40s

FACE SHAPE: pear
EYE SHAPE: basic
EYESHADOW:
highlight – shimmer beige
midtone – matte taupe
contour – shimmer golden
  brown

EYELINER: bronze
BLUSH: soft peach
LIP LINER: caramel
LIPSTICK: peachy nude
LIP GLOSS: shimmer coral

APPLICATION TIPS: Softening Linda's jawline and defining her eyes really took years off her age. She is proof that choosing the right shades can make a huge difference. Beautiful, warm shades really added life to her face and gave her a youthful glow. She is truly proof of how sculpting the face can make such a big difference.

carol, 60s

FACE SHAPE: round
EYE SHAPE: droopy
EYESHADOW:
highlight – shimmer beige
midtone – matte taupe
contour – shimmer golden
  brown

EYELINER: black
BLUSH: soft peach
LIP LINER: caramel
LIPSTICK: peachy nude
LIP GLOSS: shimmer rose

APPLICATION TIPS: Visually lifting the outer corner of Carol's eyes immediately makes her look younger. Choosing the right shades of eyeshadow also really brings out the blue in her eyes. You can see how contouring the outer edges of her face dramatically slims her face and helps accentuate her beautiful features.

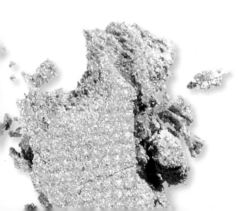

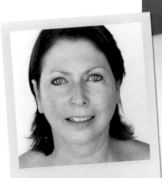

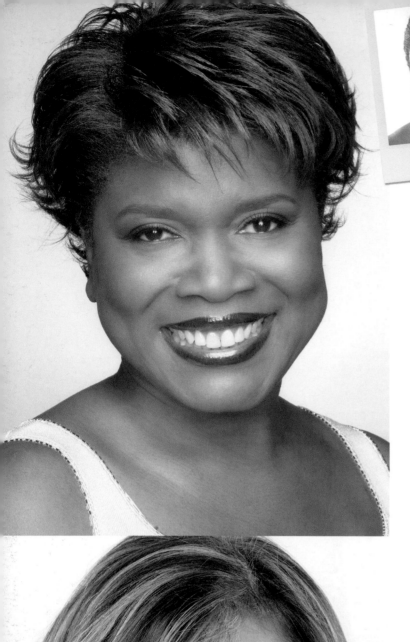

ann, 50s

FACE SHAPE: pear
EYE SHAPE: basic
EYESHADOW:

highlight – shimmer gold
midtone – matte mahogany
contour – shimmer garnet

EYELINER: black
BLUSH: soft brick
LIP LINER: soft berry
LIPSTICK: deep berry
LIP GLOSS: shimmer bronze

APPLICATION TIPS: Ann is the perfect example of how beautiful, even skin can make you look younger. By covering her dark circles and giving her skin a gorgeous glow, we took years off her age. You can also see how making the right brow color choice is paramount. I chose a shade that would soften the brow color and give her brows definition without being harsh.

tricia, 60s

FACE SHAPE: heart
EYE SHAPE: hooded
EYESHADOW:

highlight – matte nude/
    shimmer flesh
midtone – matte taupe
contour – shimmer golden
    brown

EYELINER: bronze
BLUSH: soft peach
LIP LINER: warm caramel
LIPSTICK: creamy toffee
LIP GLOSS: shimmer coral

APPLICATION TIPS: A little more definition all around really helped Tricia look younger. Curled, thick, dark lashes beautifully define her eyes. I added a big pop of color on her cheeks, first with bronzer to give her entire face a glow, then with blush on the apples of her cheeks. Adding color to Tricia's lips defines them and makes them look fuller and more youthful. Glossy lips are always sexy and young.

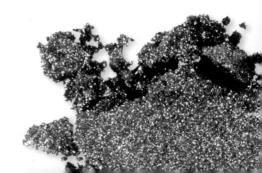

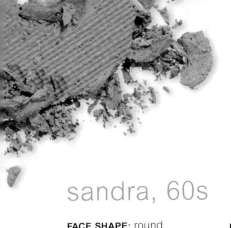

sandra, 60s

FACE SHAPE: round
EYE SHAPE: hooded
EYESHADOW:
highlight – shimmer flesh
midtone – matte taupe
contour – matte warm brown

EYELINER: dark brown
BLUSH: soft peach
LIP LINER: flesh
LIPSTICK: coral
LIP GLOSS: shimmer peach

APPLICATION TIPS: Simply covering Sandra's hyperpigmentation and broken capillaries made a huge difference and added a beautiful glow. Using eyeshadow to push back her hooded eyelids really helps open up her eyes. Defining her brows changes her whole look; they frame her eyes and giving her a youthful appearance.

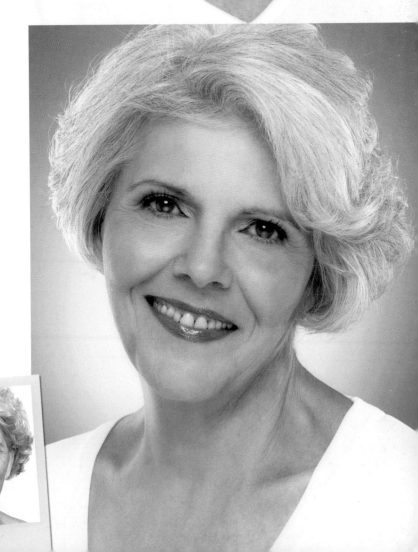

sallie, 60s

FACE SHAPE: heart
EYE SHAPE: hooded
EYESHADOW:
highlight – matte nude
midtone – matte taupe
contour – matte brown

EYELINER: bronze
BLUSH: soft peach
LIP LINER: fleshy pink
LIPSTICK: warm pink
LIP GLOSS: shimmer pink

APPLICATION TIPS: Sallie says she feels naked without lipstick, so I made sure to give her lips beautiful color. Adding definition was also helpful in making her look her most youthful. Curling her lashes and applying multiple layers of mascara really opened up her eyes. Now, if we could all just have her youthful spirit!

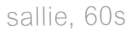

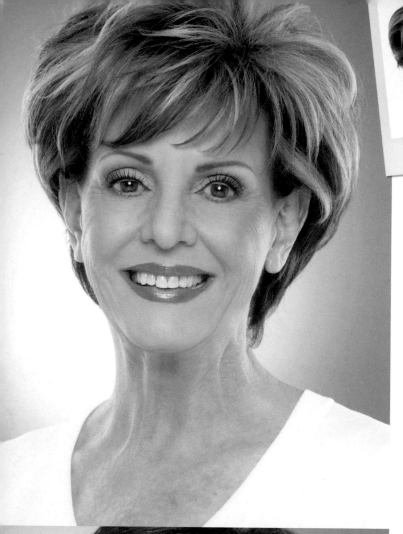

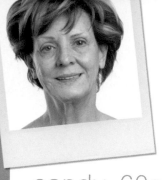

sandy, 60s

FACE SHAPE: oval
EYE SHAPE: deep-set
EYESHADOW:
highlight – matte nude
midtone – matte taupe
contour – matte warm brown

EYELINER: dark brown
BLUSH: soft peach
LIP LINER: flesh
LIPSTICK: coral
LIP GLOSS: shimmer peach

APPLICATION TIPS: Sandy is proof that fuller brows make you look younger. You can see what a difference adding definition and fullness to her brow makes. Fuller brows, a youthful glow to her skin, and she looks years younger. Never underestimate the impact of adding color and life to the face! Sandy loves full, sexy lips, and that is just what I gave her.

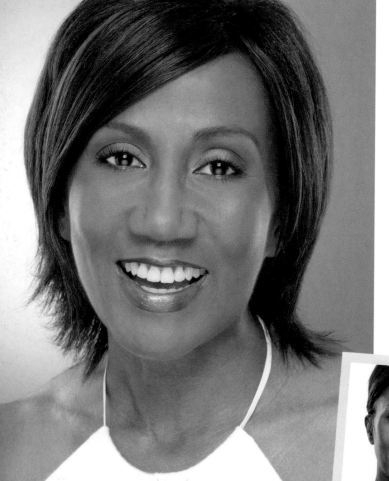

taryon, 40s

FACE SHAPE: heart
EYE SHAPE: deep-set
EYESHADOW:
highlight – shimmer gold
midtone – matte ginger
contour – shimmer garnet

EYELINER: black
BLUSH: soft brick
LIP LINER: mahogany
LIPSTICK: golden nude
LIP GLOSS: shimmer bronze

APPLICATION TIPS: Taryon just needed some soft definition to bring out her best features. She is proof that defining at the lash line can have an impact on your appearance. Thick, dark, curled lashes are a must in the quest for a youthful appearance. Notice that I did not use dark, harsh shades, just soft shades that add nice subtle definition to all of her best assets.

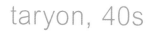

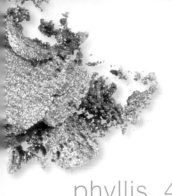

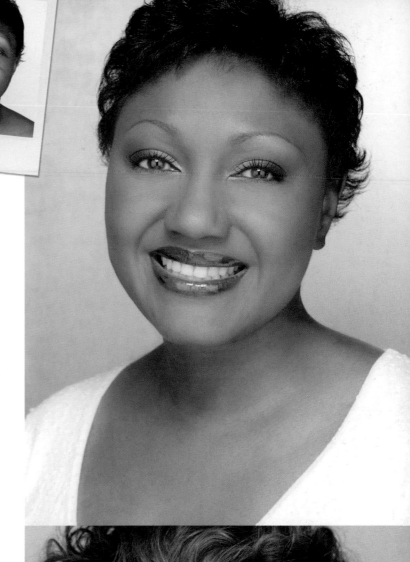

phyllis, 40s

FACE SHAPE: round
EYE SHAPE: droopy
EYESHADOW:

highlight – shimmer coral
midtone – matte mahogany
contour – matte charcoal

EYELINER: black
BLUSH: soft brick
LIP LINER: mahogany
LIPSTICK: rich raisin
LIP GLOSS: shimmer
   bronze

APPLICATION TIPS: When you look at Phyllis's "after" photo, you can see the effectiveness of correcting facial masking. It immediately makes her look younger and more beautiful. Using the perfect shades of eyeshadow, blush, and lipstick really brings it all together. Prepping Phyllis's skin before her transformation made a huge difference. Prep is a definite must!

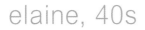

elaine, 40s

FACE SHAPE: square
EYE SHAPE: hooded
EYESHADOW:

highlight – shimmer beige
midtone – matte taupe
contour – shimmer
   chocolate

EYELINER: bronze
BLUSH: soft peach
LIP LINER: caramel
LIPSTICK: peachy nude
LIP GLOSS: creamy nude

APPLICATION TIPS: Elaine is naturally beautiful, but you can see what a difference makeup can make, even on someone who's already stunning. I love Elaine's square face—it projects such strength. You can see the difference visually pushing her eyelids back with eyeshadow makes. It really opens her eyes up and makes her look her absolute youngest.

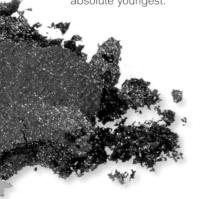

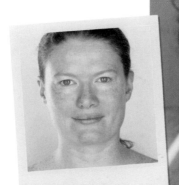

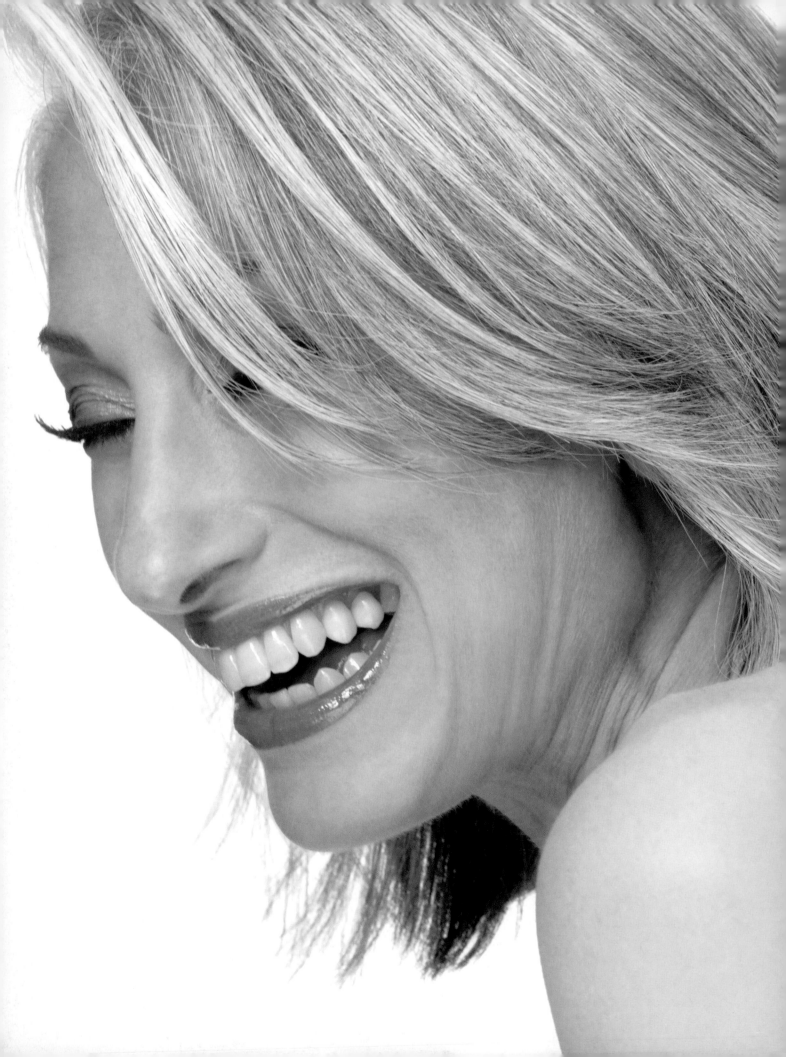

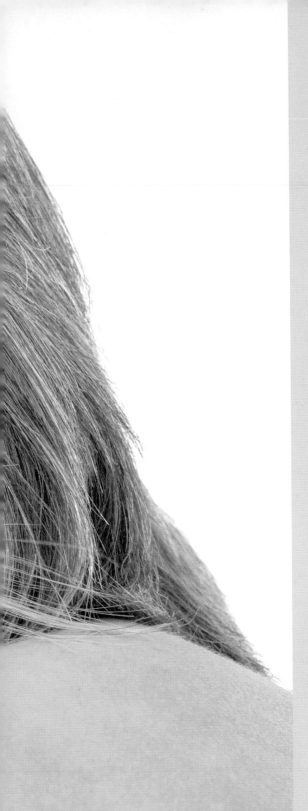

13

embracing
your true beauty

My hopes and dreams for you, now that I have armed you with the information and knowledge to look younger, are that you will use what works for you and gives you the results you desire. Remember, makeup is not rocket science! Don't let it intimidate you: If you don't get it right the first time, just wash it off and start again. Practice does make perfect! Do not expect to be a pro on your first try—keep trying, and I promise you will get the hang of it.

I hope you have enjoyed looking through the book and seeing yourself (or at least women who remind you of yourself). I have to say that I have heard it a million times, and I have to agree, "There is no such thing as an unattractive woman—just a woman who has not discovered the benefits of make-up." I know for a fact that the right color choices and application techniques—the ones I've shown you throughout this book—*will* make you look younger.

In shooting this book, I was so honored to work with so many beautiful women. A few months after the photos were finished, we sent copies to all of the models, and I received an email from one of them. The email truly puts into words why I love doing what I am blessed to be able to do.

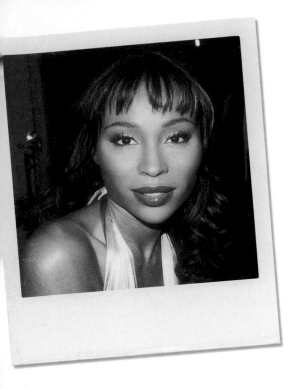

"As I look at the photo, I am reminded and amazed at how flawless my skin looks and also looked that entire day of the photo shoot! My foundation looks so much better now, because I have applied the techniques you used since that day.

"I have been a loyal fan for quite some time and have faithfully studied and applied the techniques you have shared in your books. From my experience over the years with other make-up artists, and from what I have learned from you, I've always felt I had a pretty good knowledge of how to apply my own makeup. However, after spending the day with you at the studio in Dallas, I learned several new things, including how to really perfect the application process.

"Something else I want to share… sometimes, as we look into the mirror, especially as the years pass, we can be so critical of ourselves. Robert, you have helped me to accept and appreciate myself as I am, at the age of sixty-five, wrinkles and all. I appreciate so much that you are about helping us to look and feel our very best, at *every* season of our lives! Robert, I am feeling young and vibrant again!"

Gratefully, Sandy

I'd like to leave you with one last thought. Please, do not expect or try erase what makes you your own unique self. Instead, embrace what makes you special. You can be and are beautiful; you just need to embrace your personal beauty. Use your makeup to enhance what you love about your face. Remember, beauty comes from within, and your outward beauty is an expression of your inner beauty. Love and embrace who you are, today and every day!

about the author

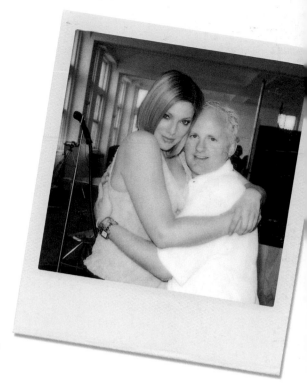

robert jones is the founder and president of robert jones beauty (www.robertjonesbeauty.com). Born and raised in Houston, he is a well-known hair and makeup artist with more than twenty years of experience. His clients include companies such as Neiman Marcus, Mary Kay Cosmetics, Watters and Watters, Bergdorf Goodman, Saks Fifth Avenue, Bloomingdales, Lord & Taylor, Olay, Avon, Nexxus, Fossil, Michelle Watches, and Levi's; magazines such as *Marie Claire, Elle, Allure, Jane, InStyle, Glamour, Brides Magazine, Elegant Bride, Shape,* and *Life and Style*; and celebrities such as Delta Burke, Diahann Carroll, Sheryl Crowe, LeAnn Rimes, Carol Channing, the Dixie Chicks, Bridget Moynahan, and many, many others.

Robert believes he fell into his makeup art with a little heavenly guidance. When he was young, he obtained a scholarship from the Museum of Fine Arts in Texas. Surrounded by many young talents, he began to believe his paintings were not deep and creative enough, and decided to instead explore and pursue an interest in acting. Later, he found a way to merge the two interests into a highly successful career as a makeup artist.

Today, Robert travels to five cities a month, giving makeup demonstrations to thousands of women across the United States. He also has his own signature line of best-selling brushes and makeup tools, as well as a forthcoming makeup line. His previous books, *Makeup Makeovers* and *Makeup Makeovers: Weddings*, have sold more than 100,000 copies.

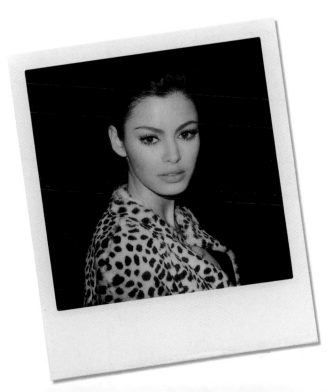

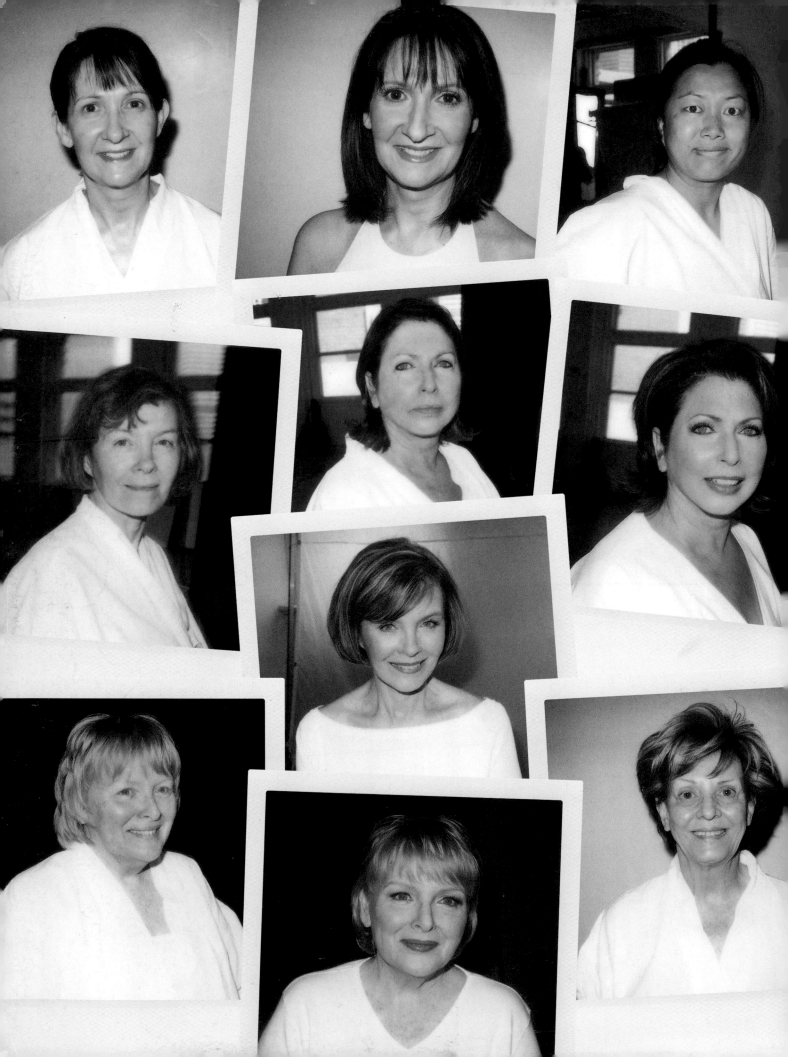

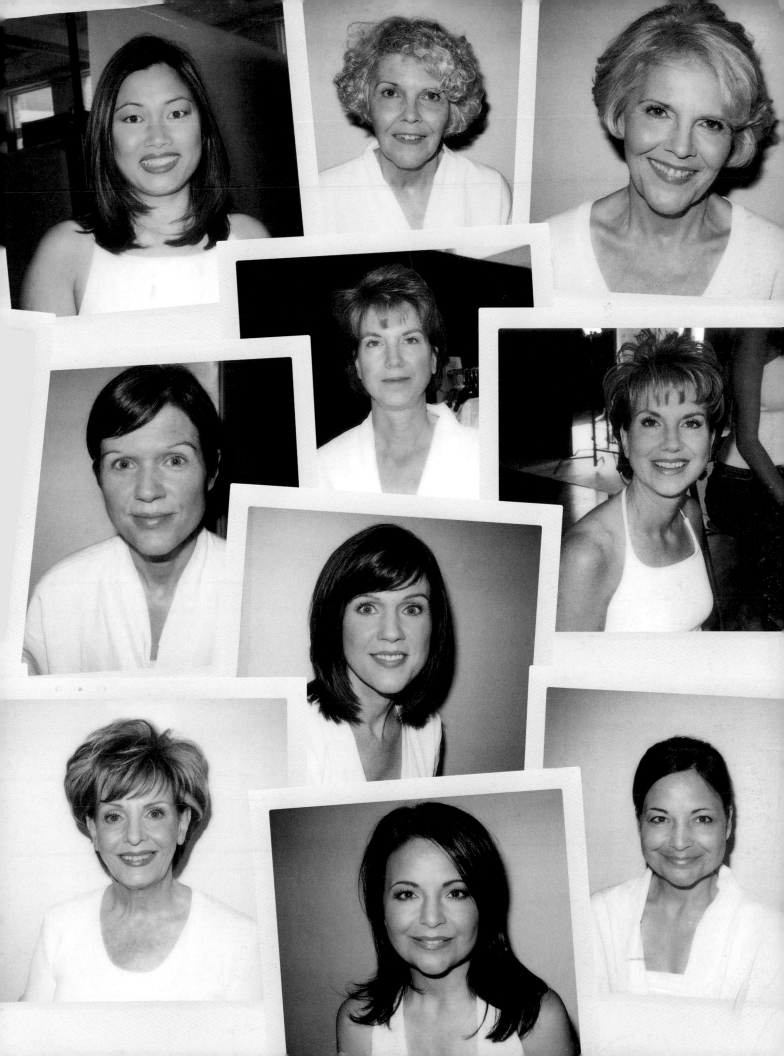